NEW REVISED EDITION

CATHERINE KALAMIS
WITH SIOFRA BRENNAN

WOMEN
without
SEX

THE TRUTH
ABOUT FEMALE
SEXUAL
PROBLEMS

SELF-HELP DIRECT

www.selfhelpdirect.com

Design: Mitchell Davies & Michael Crozier/Design Unlimited
Illustration: Michael Roscoe

Published by Self-Help Direct Publishing, PO Box 9085, London, N12 8ED
First edition 1999
Second edition 2003
Third edition 2007

ISBN 978 1 900461 35 1

For more copies of this book, please send a £12.95 cheque/postal order per book
(overseas sales €25/US$25 per book, postage & packing free) to the address
below. Make cheques payable to Self-Help Direct.

Self-Help Direct Publishing
PO BOX 9035,
London, N12 8ED

---

*The Sexual Dysfunction Association (formerly the Impotence Association),
PO Box 10296, London, SW17 9WH (tel: 020 8767 7791 www.impotence.org.uk)*

Relate, Herbert Gray College, Little Church Street, Rugby CV21 3AP (tel: 01788 573241)

introduction..7

1   how does it feel?...10
how to recognise FSD; the research so far

2   what is female sexual dysfunction?...............................18
sexual arousal; young and old; how research is conducted; lack of sexual
drive; female sexual function questionnaire

3   sex and physiology...41
key elements of physical and sexual arousal; the P-spot and the G-spot;
diseases and disorders; sex hormones;

4   sex and the mind..60
psychosexual counselling; psychological problems; loss of sexual
feelings; sex therapy

5   sex and the menopause..71
pyschological influences; physical and sexual changes; HRT; sensual
exercises; love and getter older

6   painful sex..89
common causes; key symptoms; vaginismus; self care; vulval complaints

7   trial and tribulations—new treatments........................98
drugs; patches, gels and creams; nasal sprays; tablets; herbs; gadgets; surgery

8   testosterone – the hormone of desire?.....................112
treatments; tests

9   looking after yourself..117
improving your health; exercise; health problems; alcohol

10   the happiness factor...121
self-worth and self-esteem; food for love; sex supplements; pelvic floor
exercises; massage, self-stimulation

11   adjustments to your sex life...................................131
sex after childbirth; sex and modern life

12   fantasy and lovemaking techniques.........................137
useful aids; masturbation; sexual techniques

Foreword

We live in an age where we are given the impression that good sex is ours for the asking. If we're not getting it, then there's something wrong — and we tend to think we're the ones who are 'abnormal'. Yet most people experience difficulties in their sex lives at some time. In the early days of any new sexual relationship, desire is high. People can't get enough of each other. During sex and orgasm dopamine levels soar[1]. Brain scans of people having an orgasm resemble the scans of a heroin rush[2]. After orgasm, dopamine plummets, prolactin soars and androgen receptor activity decreases for up to a week. Rises in prolactin act as a sexual satiation mechanism[3].

We are at the mercy of our hormones. But they are not the only factors affecting our sexual behaviour. The circumstances in which we live and work, our family life stage, our personalities and emotional resources all have an impact. When you've been up in the night feeding a baby and wrestling with a toddler during the day, sex is the last thing on your mind. In order to feel like sex, many women need to feel good about themselves, their children, their relationship with their partner, their extended family, their job, their home, etc. Whereas if their partners feel uneasy about these things, then they may need sex all the more to help them to cope. What a recipe for disaster! It's a wonder any couples make it after the first few years!

Yet many couples do continue to make love throughout their relationships. Sex remains a way of expressing intimacy, affection, healing and fun. If couples are unable to have intercourse, they miss this part of their relationship, however infrequent their lovemaking has become. It is a real loss.

For women in past generations, sex was (and currently in some cultures, still is) seen as a duty. The law has been slow to criminalise sexual assault in intimate relationships, challenging the notion of a man's 'conjugal rights'. But fortunately the Victorian adage, to 'lie back and think of England' has become a joke. Many women, as a matter of principle, will not consider sex unless they are 'in the mood'. However, recent research by Rosemary Basson[4] has resulted in the Intimacy-based Model of Female Sexual Response. It is clear that many women may not be 'in the mood' for sex, but know that once love-making begins, they will probably become aroused and their desire is awakened. An important factor in this is the level of intimacy in the relationship at the time. Some women report that for the sake of the relationship, they are willing to make love, but do not see this as a 'duty'.

It used to be thought that the reasons for sexual difficulties were either psychological or physical. It is now widely recognised that this is too simplistic.

Whenever there are physical conditions affecting sexual functioning, there are always psychological factors impacting on the situation as well.

Some years ago Laura and Paul came to see me for sex therapy at Relate. The couple had not had intercourse for four years, following the birth of their last child, Sam, who was severely disabled. They had even stopped showing any physical affection for each other, but said they still loved each other. The birth of the child had been physically and emotionally traumatic. The family had just moved away from their first home and Paul had to work long hours, often away from home. The first time they attempted intercourse after Sam's birth, it was painful for Laura. The pain was still there whenever they attempted intercourse after that, and so they stopped trying. I asked Laura to have another physical check, just in case, but her gynaecologist confirmed that there was nothing organically wrong. Laura and Paul hadn't been able to talk about any of this together — it had all been too stressful. An important part of the therapy was encouraging them to share all this. The sex therapy exercises I set them were very useful, but without sharing their feelings, I doubt we would have progressed. At the end of their treatment, their relationship as well as their sex lives had healed.

The information in this book will be extremely useful to anyone needing help with their sexual problems. It will also be useful for therapists and health professionals to recommend to their clients.

Christine Lacy — Practice and Supervision Consultant, Relate Institute.

References

[1]Putnam, S.K., Du, J., Sato, S., & Hull, E.M. (2001) Testosterone restoration of copulatory behavior correlates with medial preoptic dopamine release in castrated male rats. *Hormones and Behavior* 2001 May; 39(3): 216-24

[2]Holstege, G., Georgiadis, J.R., Paans, A.M.J., Meiners, L.C., van der Graaf, F.H.C.E., 4 & Reinders, A.A.T.S. (2003). Brain activation during human male ejaculation. *The Journal of Neuroscience*, 23(27): 9185-9193

[3]Kruger (2003) "Effects of acute prolactin manipulation on sexual drive and function in males" *Journal of Endocrinology*, Vol 179, Issue 3, 357-365

[4]Basson *et al*, (2003), Definitions of women's sexual disorder reconsidered: advocating expansion and revision in *Journal of Psychosomatic Obstetric and Gynaecology*. 2003; 24(4): 221-9., Lippincott, Williams & Wilkins, Core

Preface

When the second edition of this book was published in 2003, attitudes to female sexual dysfunction (FSD) were changing. The Impotence Association had just changed its name to the Sexual Dysfunction Association (SDA) to reflect the numbers of women contacting them. Organisations such as the SDA and sex counsellors were beginning to recognise that FSD can have biological as well as psychological causes.

At the time new drugs to treat FSD were expected to be available in the UK within months. Certainly, nobody believed that a single magic pill or potion would cure the broad range of sexual problems experienced by women. However, drug treatments for specific problems, which would benefit certain groups of women, have largely failed to materialise as anticipated.

Pharmaceutical companies have discovered that FSD is much more complex than erectile dysfunction in men. A woman's ability to enjoy sex depends on a number of factors, many of them psychological. Unlike with men, arousal and desire are separate and do not necessarily occur at the same time for women. Creating a treatment that merely increases a woman's physical arousal has not proved to be an adequate solution to sexual problems. Clinicians still expect that drugs will eventually be launched but their development is taking longer than first expected.

Women have been taking part in clinical trials and potential treatments have received widespread media coverage. As a result, there is now a greater awareness of sexual dysfunction than there was 10 years ago. Women have spoken openly in the press about their complete lack of sexual desire. Magazines aimed at women in their 20s and 30s have acknowledged that FSD is a problem affecting their readers and not just older women who have been through the menopause.

Alongside this increased awareness is a denial that FSD even exists. Campaigners who accuse pharmaceutical companies of 'disease mongering' have seized on the failure to find suitable drug treatments as evidence of this.

Yet, research suggests that up to 43% of women are experiencing sexual difficulties at any one time. That means that there are many women who are desperately seeking information and help. That is what I hope the third edition of this book will provide.

Siofra Brennan
London, March 2007

Introduction

*L*osing your sexuality is like losing a language. When you don't have a satisfactory sex life then you lose an act of communication. That is the view of 30-year-old Anna who suffers from female sexual dysfunction. She is not alone. One independent market analyst has estimated that around 90 million women across Europe, Japan and the US are affected by some form of FSD[1]. The baseline for the statistical evidence comes from research derived from the US National Health and Social Life Survey compiled by a consortium of private foundations and without drug company support.

Prof. Edward Laumann, professor of sociology and Fellow of the American Association for the Advancement of Science, reported a preliminary analysis of this data for a chapter of his book (*The Social Organisation of Sexuality*[2]) in 1994 – at least four years before the advent of Viagra. The same data was used in a paper for the *Journal of American Medical Association*[3]. He found that 43% of women had suffered a sexual dysfunction of some duration in the previous 12 months.

He said: 'I do not believe that the figure of 43% . . . is empirically wrong or in any way exaggerates the problem. It is in fact self-reported by a representative sample of women living in the US. It is likely to be an under-estimate since it is reasonable to assume that some people were reluctant to report such a condition.'

Prof. Laumann served as a member of a scientific advisory panel for Pfizer, the drug company, but said he has never had any grant to support his own research, which is data collection, from a drug company. 'When I have helped analyse data for Pfizer I have always explicitly identified myself as a consultant on the project.'

He has replicated this work in a number of other countries including a sample study in China with 'essentially the same results'. He makes it clear that female sexual dysfunction has a number of causes – some of which may respond to medication, perhaps most effectively when combined with attention to other parts of a woman's life such as relationships, and 'life circumstances'.

However, even an editorial in the respected *British Medical Journal*[4] has questioned the existence of FSD by posing a number of questions. 'Is a new disorder being identified to meet unmet needs or build markets for new medications?'

So is there an unmet need for attention or are the pharmaceutical giants just exploiting the fears of women? My belief is that FSD is real. Women are coming forward, some after years of silence, and their stories of sexual dysfunction ring true. Once, women may have accepted a life without sex. But society has changed and women are no longer prepared to tolerate such an important gap in their lives. In the past, women often believed no one else had the same problems, or that what they felt was a depressing part of getting old. They feared their partners thought they no longer loved them, or suspected them of being unfaithful because they no longer wanted sex.

And what relief they felt when they were told they were not alone or odd, that it had nothing to do with ageing – that women can be enjoying sex into their 80s or beyond if that is what they want.

The problem with female sexual dysfunction at present is understanding 'what is normal?' In simple terms 'normal' is what feels right for you, and your partner. When things don't feel 'right', when sex fails to feature in your life even though you want it to, and when this loss affects your relationships, then you may be experiencing a dysfunction or a sexual disinterest that needs addressing. I explain this in more detail later on and offer a questionnaire which should help to establish whether you have any form of FSD. What is certainly true is that there are many, many women around the world who apparently have deeply unsatisfactory sex lives. It is also true that for many women an admission of this remains taboo.

If you suffer sexual dysfunction or disappointment it can go to the heart and soul of your life and your relationships. Knowing you are not a freak, frigid or 'losing it' is vital for psychological well-being.

Since the first edition of this book was published in 1999 there has been a greater acceptance and recognition of FSD – and it's not all driven by the drug companies whatever the critics may say. Most appointments with Relate's sexual therapy services are now made by women, and in 2002 50 lone women made contact. Women have been ringing the Sexual Dysfunction Association – as the only public point of contact – in their hundreds. If FSD did not exist women would be boycotting drugs trials. Instead, they want to join them. However, I believe that treatment for women will come about in a different way to Viagra for men. I don't believe in a universal panacea – one pink 'lifestyle' pill that will correct a faulty relationship and make sex better.

I believe a small range of products with different actions will eventually become available to help women who have become distressed by physiological problems that have been determined by medical tests and questionnaires. How women choose to deal with their sexual problems is highly individual but surely it is better to have some options rather than none? Women don't want to be 'medicalised' – but if they are experiencing a problem which is causing them anguish, then what is wrong with an expectation of help and treatment?

After years of living in the shadows we now know that women – just like men – can suffer from an inability to enjoy, desire, or participate in sex with their partner when they want to because of a disorder.

The burning questions still remain: how do women recover? Can they? How do they access help? What is available? Could any of the treatments work for them? This book aims to provide some answers. One thing is certain. FSD has entered people's consciousness. And it's not going away.

References

[1]Datamonitor Executive Summary by Datamonitor Healthcare from Strategic Perspectives: Female Sexual Dysfunction. Are physicians and patients ready for a female Viagra? August 2002, Datamonitor Europe, Charles House, 108-110 Finchley Road, London NW3 5JJ (tel: 020 7675 7000).

[2]Laumann, E. O., *et al*. The Social Organisation of Sexuality: Sexual Practices in the United States. University of Chicago Press 1994 (paperback, UCP 2001).

[3]Laumann, E. O., Paik, A., Rosen, R. C. Sexual dysfunction in the United States: prevalence and predictors. *Journal of American Medical Association* 1999. **281**: 1174, 537-544.

[4]*British Medical Journal* 2003. **326**: 45-47.

1

how does it feel?

You may have wondered why you don't have that 'natural instinct' for sex other women describe. Or why you've lost the sexual spark you used to enjoy in your partner's presence. You may have questioned your own sexual identity because you find it difficult, or impossible, to become sexually aroused.

You may have gone through sexual therapy or counselling and perhaps tried HRT. Doctors, possibly partners, might have told you that what you are experiencing, however distressing, is 'all part of the ageing process', a 'natural consequence' of having a baby or changing your lifestyle, or simply suggested that 'this is normal for you'.

If you are suffering from female sexual dysfunction you may never have had an orgasm, or felt sexually excited. You may once have enjoyed sex but now suffer unexplained pain on intercourse, a distressing lack of lubrication, a complete loss of genital sensation.

Despite these discomforts you may succumb to sex for the emotional reward of the closeness or companionship of a partner but you may be beginning to dread the act.

You may struggle with what you think is a unique flaw in your sexuality, one that strikes at the heart of your relationships. But you cope by locking the problem away in the back of your mind, telling yourself: 'Nothing can be done so I'll put my energies into something else, like the children, or career.'

Your partner may have been expressing some dissatisfaction too – because you never feel like initiating sex. (Years ago men expected sexually passive partners. Now they expect women to initiate sex, too, and can complain when this does not happen).

Quick questions: How to recognise FSD

- Do you have less sexual desire than before and does this worry you?
- Do you have a burning sensation in the vagina during intercourse?
- Does it hurt when you have sex – and does your vagina remain dry?
- Are you worried that you can no longer achieve orgasm as you used to?
- Have you noticed a decrease in sensation in the genital area and clitoris?
- Do you desire sex less even though you love your partner and does this feels like a problem you want to change?
- Are you distressed about any aspect of your sex life?

If you answer yes to any of these questions then it might help to talk to a specialist with an interest in sexual medicine.

The research

This revised edition examines in detail the deep well of unhappiness that exists among women whose sexual problems have not been fully recognised. Studies into the impact of sexual problems on the sex lives of women have involved personal interviews with women in numerous countries. These interviews uncovered the misery sexual problems cause women and the effects on their partners, their relationships and their lifestyles. One of these studies was conducted by Dr Frances Quirk, a psychologist and a senior clinician with Pfizer. She suffered unexpectedly from FSD herself, as a result of a thyroid disorder, so understands the feeling of loss, shock and distress experienced by women. Her story appears on page 55.

Dr Quirk has used her research to report on the impact of sexual difficulties on the quality of life of modern women – focusing particularly on the social, physical, emotional and psychological consequences of sexual problems. Details of these findings are to be found later in this book.

Her work, and research by specialists with an interest and growing expertise in sexual medicine both in the UK and America, are already providing the foundation for innovative clinical approaches to female sexual problems. The diagnostic 'bibles' used by clinicians are changing to take into account new information about women's sexual response, sexuality and sexual difficulties.

Women of today – part of the Pill generation – want answers if their sex life deteriorates. They believe that men have been helped with Viagra. Now women are insisting: 'What about us?'

And there is good reason. What is new about FSD is the firm belief, backed by science, that a high proportion of female sexual problems have a physical, biological cause.

For example, a woman who is unable to have an orgasm or has difficulty in feeling sexy may have a condition recently identified as clitoral insufficiency that is due to a poor or interrupted flow of blood to the erectile tissue of the clitoris. Or she may have a hormonal abnormality, which puts the brakes on sexual drive. An inability to lubricate might be triggered by specific impairments of the arterial circulation into the vagina, which interferes with the normal vascular processes required for lovemaking.

There are other causes of FSD, just as there are for erectile dysfunction in men – and these are linked with diabetes, multiple sclerosis (MS), high cholesterol levels, a narrowing of the arteries and heart disease, certain prescription drugs (particularly some anti-depressants), blood vessel or nerve damage from pelvic or abdominal surgery such as hysterectomies, some gynaecological cancer treatments, breast cancer, childbirth, and hormonal irregularities. There are a host of conditions associated with vulval disorders. Painful sex is a problem for many women of all ages due to a range of conditions that may be psychological or physiological. And research indicates clearly that the biggest problems for women are 'loss of desire' (the Laumann report from the US found that 33% of 1,749 women picked at random had this problem) and 'an inability, or difficulty, in becoming sexually aroused'.

The problem with the FSD story is that it takes many twists and turns. The key is understanding your particular problem – or problems – and then combining treatment or self-help action. FSD problems may be interlinked and may have several causes – possibly triggered by hormone imbalances or an underlying inefficiency of vital chemical or neurological messengers which all play a part in the female sexual response sending signals from the brain to the genitals.

Some desire problems may be connected with psychological 'blocks': if there is pain on intercourse due to an underlying physiological problem then you are likely to anticipate pain next time and so start a vicious cycle. You may need help not only to remove the physical 'stumbling block' but also to overcome the 'pain barrier'.

Physiological female sexual arousal difficulties have a direct parallel with erectile dysfunction in men because both conditions are caused by blood flow problems. (This condition was called female impotence before being taken under the all-encompassing umbrella of FSD.)

Since these sexual difficulties were acknowledged as medical conditions, the race has been on among leading pharmaceutical companies to develop drugs that will be licensed for the treatment of FSD. Procter & Gamble's testosterone patch Intrinsa has been licensed in Europe for women up whose ovaries have been removed. At the time of writing the patch had just been launched in the UK. Intrinsa is now available on prescription to women under 60 who are surgically menopausal and have diagnosed sexual problems, making it the first licensed drug treatment for hypoactive sexual desire disorder. Details of Intrinsa and other potential medications can be found in chapter seven. However, as yet no drug has been licensed to treat the broad spectrum of female sexual dysfunctions.

Despite some physiological similarities, there is, however, a fundamental difference which makes the female equivalent of sexual arousal problems more complex to manage medically than male impotence or erectile dysfunction. On the whole, a woman's emotional needs also have to be met for good sex to occur – there has to be a psychological bonding. Women often engage in sex just to be close to their partners, while men often seek sex just for the pleasure they derive from the act itself.

Sex for a woman tends to be an expression of the relationship – and if a man cannot stimulate a woman in the right way, nor respond to or understand her individual needs, she may suffer sexually. Research indicates that an older women may need to re-evaluate her sex life: after years together couples may need to find different ways of stimulating each other in order to avoid sex becoming a bind, or even dwindling to a halt.

One woman in her 50s said of her sexual difficulty: 'I've never really considered myself as getting old and now I can see different things happening to my body. The sex is not as often as it used to be so when we do have sex, I use a lubricant. After the lubrication and penetration then comes the dryness. It's not a comfortable feeling. At first I felt very down, I felt like something was missing. Maybe I felt like I wasn't complete. The first time it happened I could not stand the penetration and I asked him to stop and I could see the hurt in his face.'

Since the first edition of this book in 1999 the Sexual Dysfunction Association has received thousands of calls from women asking for information about their sexual problems. Drug companies have been contacted by women wanting to take part in trials. Women have expressed relief that someone is prepared to listen to them, said Dr Mitra Boolell, former Pfizer clinical team leader in Sandwich, Kent.

Dr Boolell said: 'Health professionals need to recognise that sexual health has a huge impact on other aspects of life and on quality of life. The medical profession tends not to ask questions about sexual health matters – it is embarrassing to bring them up. But this is something I believe will change.'

How many women are affected – the research so far.

A report[1] compiled in 2001 showed that in the last 10 years there have been 52 studies on sexual dysfunction in men and women. Few were large-scale studies, but the researchers extracted information from numerous smaller ones. When they compared data from different studies they found the following range of women reporting problems.

- Orgasm: 4-24%
- Arousal: 8-19%
- Low libido: 5-46%
- Painful sex: 9-21%

In 1998 a GP-based UK survey[2] found that 41% of female respondents reported an ongoing sexual problem with 68% of women reporting a sexual problem at some time in their lives. The most common complaint was vaginal dryness and orgasm problems. This compared to the 'baseline' Laumann report of 1999, which suggested 43% of American women had experienced a sexual dysfunction at some time in the previous year. In 1999 a Swedish survey[3] among 2,810 men and women aged 18 to 74 found that 14% of women had impaired sexual desire; 15% had decreased sexual interest; 8% had lubrication difficulties; 10% had orgasm problems; and 4% complained of painful sex.

There are now more than 50 doctors around the UK with an interest in FSD. International symposiums – which have been held in such diverse locations as Vancouver, London and Hamburg – are helping to spread the word. New treatments will undoubtedly become available over the next five years. Some are already with us. Sex therapy is available for women, and drugs to treat specific physiological problems preventing women from enjoying a fulfilling sex life have been launched. Gadgets designed specifically to stimulate the clitoris are on the market now.

All this has to be set against a background of cultural and social change: sexual problems are coming out of the closet, into the open. The question: 'How many times a week is normal?' is being replaced with 'Why am I missing out on any joyful sex?' followed by 'What can be done to help?' Meanwhile, specialists in sexual medicine who had been working on solutions for male erectile dysfunction (ED) problems have turned their attention to women, driven by the desire of pharmaceutical companies to understand the new market place. Some people decry this as medicalisation of FSD. Surely it can only be good that FSD is now out there alongside ED? It exists, it is a problem, and hopefully it can be resolved whether by natural means, through

---

WHY NOW?

Research into women's sexual problems is still about a decade behind the research into male impotence. There is a growing demand for help and information from women themselves who are now ready to speak up about their problems which range from never having experienced an orgasm to a complete loss of desire or drive, to avoiding sex with their partner even though that partner may be deeply loved.

Sex today is seen as an important part of a woman's overall health and well-being. There is no doubt that a good sex life enhances quality of life and, according to Dr Beverly Whipple who rediscovered the G-spot, sex also 'fosters personal growth and contributes to human fulfillment'. She writes: 'When the term sexuality is viewed holistically it refers to the totality of being. It refers to human qualities and not just to the genitals and their functions. It includes all the qualities – biological, psychological, emotional, cultural, social and spiritual – that makes people who they are.' In essence, woman today should expect to have a good sex life and be able to receive help if they are not having one. This is a fundamentally new and different approach to the most private and intimate part of our lives. In the past women have tended to complain about the more 'subjective' qualities of the sexual experience rather than specific physiological difficulties, says Dr John Bancroft, head of the Kinsey Institute in the US. The most common complaints have been loss of sexual

counselling, or with the help of a pill, patch, cream or device.

Sexual dysfunctions in women are now receiving attention and funding. But there is still a long way to go and treatment is patchy: there are gynaecologists who are interested in FSD, as well as genito-urinary specialists and GPs, clinical psychologists, even skin specialists. All these different strands can be confusing.

Where do you go for help? It is time doctors joined together to form a common approach and methodology.

Women's sexual problems have largely been ignored in the past, because women are far more difficult to investigate. Research indicates that while men want a 'quick fix' for their problems, women want to increase their sexual desire in order to improve their relationships: this involves a more complex combination of mechanical and psychological factors. But as sexual medicine advances, better ways have been found to measure female sexual response and so discoveries are being made about women and for women. This is coupled with a demand for more information from women themselves — and the acknowledgment that these problems really do exist and they do affect quality of life.

Prof. Laumann said of his ground-breaking work: 'The results . . . indicate that sexual problems are widespread in society and are influenced by both health-related and psychosocial factors. The role of the latter implies that stress inducing events due to either individual or social sources, can affect sexual functioning in both men and women. With the strong association between sexual dysfunction and impaired quality of life, this problem warrants recognition as a significant public health concern.'

---

desire, loss of enjoyment of sex, difficulty in reaching orgasm, and pain during intercourse. The problem until recently was how to evaluate sexual arousal in a woman in laboratory conditions. Now there is a range of instruments which can be used to measure blood movement and blood volume in the vagina, indicating levels of physiological arousal – just as an erect penis indicates arousal in a man. This clinical work is helping to provide some answers on women's physiological response. New questionnaires have also been devised and one of them is now included in this book. This form of 'self-evaluation' is now a recognised way of measuring FSD, which can be influenced by clinical conditions or invasive laboratory techniques. The problem with female sexual dysfunction is that there is no single cause: there are many. The

challenge for health professionals and drug companies is to identify the different 'types' and produce a range of potential treatments to suit. Since this book was first published the subject has become much clearer but there is still a long way to go in terms of informing women, then offering them hope of a solution.

Women, deluged with information about progress on male impotence, are coming forward to say they, too, have a fundamental problem that affects their health and lifestyle. Rather than put up with it as their mother's generation might have preferred to do, possibly encouraged by their embarrassed husbands or medical advisers, today's women are asking in no uncertain terms what their doctors are going to do about it.

Viagra has not proven to be the great solution it was considered to be for men. Pfizer suspended its trials of the drug on women in after eight years of testing. In trials the drug was found to create outward signs of arousal in many women, but it had little effect on their willingness, or desire, to have sex. Pfizer has now turned its attention to investigating drugs that affect women's brain chemistry.

In the absence of any licensed drug to treat FSD, there are other answers to sexual problems. This book examines some of them:

- the importance of understanding how and where women can be sexually stimulated: new information about erogenous zones.
- the importance of exercise in stimulating sexual response.
- why watching a thrilling movie or drinking a cup of strong coffee may boost low sexual desire by stimulating the sympathetic nervous system.
- how different lovemaking techniques and breathing exercises may help
- why testosterone may be the answer to some women's sexual problems: success in the UK and Australia with testosterone implants.
- the influence of oestrogen-rich foods, a change in diet, and use of herbs and aphrodisiacs and Chinese medicine.
- how a small hand-held device has become the first recognised treatment for FSD in the world.
- how to talk to your doctor and avoid embarrassment: where to find a sympathetic specialist.

Extraordinary as it may sound, one of the spin-offs from this fresh approach to female sexual dysfunction is a greater understanding of female physiology. Another is a deeper awareness of the complexities of female sexual arousal and female sexuality. Some of it is so far-reaching that anatomy text books will have to be re-written. This is explored in a special section of this book, which explains the known elements of female sexual arousal, recent discoveries concerning the clitoris and the role of the urethra, which is surrounded by 'erectile tissue' and effectively becomes a sexual organ in women.

Summary
Specialists working in the field of sexual medicine agree that female sexual dysfunction exists, but that it tends to be more complex than male impotence and contrary to popular opinion affects younger women as well as older. Allegations have been levelled at pharmaceutical companies for making up and 'medicalising' the condition. There is another side of the coin, according to supporters of groups campaigning to stop the medicalisation of women's sexual health.

Their view is that FSD has as much to do with the way women view their bodies, and themselves; social factors such as confidence levels; how respected they feel; stress in their daily lives; age and education level; the quality of their sexual education; economic standing; their degree of comfort with their bodies; what medications they are taking; and their relationship satisfaction.

'Women need to feel safety and respect to maintain their initial sexual attraction, they need to feel the burdens of life are shared (for example, child care, elder care, and domestic chores), and they need to feel their partner is interested in them as a human being – that's the part that's often missing,' according to US organisation, FSD Alert.

Further reading and information
Kinsey Institute – Information Services
Morrison Hall 302, 1165 East Third Street, Bloomington, IN 47405, USA
Tel 812/855-7686 fax 812/855-8277
www.kinseyinstitute.org
Kinsey@indiana.edu

References
[1]Simons and Carey, Prevalence of Sexual Dysfunctions: Results from a Decade of Research, Plenium Publishing, 2001.
[2]Dunn, K. M., Croft, P. R., Hackett, G. I. Sexual problems: a study of the prevalence and need for health care in the general population. *Family Practice* 1998; **15**: 519-24.
[3]Fugl-Meyer, A. R., Fugl-Meyer, K. S. Sexual Disabilities, problems and satisfaction in 18-64-year-old Swedes, 1999, *Scandinavian Journal of Sexology*; **3**: 79-105.

2

what is female sexual dysfunction?

'I feel I have lost my femininity and womanhood. I can't have sex and I am unable to have children. It's left me feeling empty.'
Susan, aged 54.

Traditionally, women have remained quiet about their sexual problems, putting up with them without too much complaint. Consequently women with sexual problems were simply not taken seriously or frequently labelled 'frigid'. There is now an awareness that women do experience sexual dysfunction but it is still not widely understood that this can happen as a direct result of disease, or arterial, neurological or hormonal problems.

However some doctors say that when it comes to understanding women's sexual problems, we are only at the stage we were with male impotence 15 years ago. And there are health professionals who still don't know how to react to women's concerns. Datamonitor Healthcare conducted an analysis of the potential 'market' for women patients with FSD for the drug industry. An executive summary of the research commented:

'Even when patients do seek help, physicians may downplay their concerns, whether out of their own embarrassment, lack of awareness of the availability of services and concerns regarding the potential costs, all serving as barriers to presentation. It is clear that there is an immense need within FSD not only for effective well-tolerated pharmacological therapies, but more fundamentally improved education for physicians and patients.'

Female sexual dysfunction has not been considered by the medical profession as a serious enough disorder to warrant much time or energy – until now, when the implications for possible new treatments are so clearly on the horizon. And there is still a haziness surrounding classification – even doctors are confused as to whether FSD is physical or psychological, multiple or separate conditions, or whether it is a condition that exists at all.

Only one in four women affected make it to a doctor and just a small percentage currently get the help they deserve, according to Datamonitor Healthcare. These findings are backed up by a survey conducted by Dr John Dean, a GP specialist in sexual medicine, who sent questionnaires to 600 family doctors in two areas of the UK. The GPs reported that 'few women seek advice from them'; there was particular confusion about the term 'arousal disorder'; and, confirming what many women patients suspect, few of the doctors said they felt confident in assessing and managing FSD. Dr Dean concluded that 'UK family physicians require specific training to meet the needs of women with FSD'.

Whether doctors like it or not, women do suffer from sexual problems, although many women accept the situation without complaint. Prof. Laumann – whose earlier work revealed the extent of FSD in America – is the joint author of a global study[1] of sexual attitude and behaviour which investigates attitudes, beliefs, and behaviour regarding sex, intimacy, and relationships. The survey on sexual attitudes involved 14,714 men and 12,786 women aged between 40 and 80 in 30 countries was presented at an international conference in Canada in October 2002 (see page 70)

Prof. Laumann concluded that FSD conditions affect women regardless of age: in other words, they are not 'menopausal' issues. He said: 'Physical factors associated with aging did not appear to consistently influence the likelihood of sexual dysfunction. Social and psychological factors appear to have much greater impact.'

However, since the last edition of this book in 2003, the Campaign for a New View of Women's Sexual Problems has been gathering force. New View held its second conference in Montreal in 2005. Leonore Tiefer, clinical associate professor of psychiatry at the New York University School of Medicine, is at the forefront of the campaign, which accuses drug companies of 'disease mongering'. In other words, manufacturing a disease so that they can sell the drugs to treat it.

In an article published in the *Journal of the Public Library of Science* in 2006, Tiefer says that sexual life has become vulnerable to disease mongering for two main reasons.

'A long history of social and political control of sexual expression created reservoirs of shame and ignorance that make it difficult for many people to understand sexual satisfaction or cope with sexual problems in rational ways,' she said. 'Secondly, popular culture has greatly inflated public expectations about sexual function and the importance of sex to personal and relationship satisfaction.'

She points out how after Pfizer's failure to prove that Viagra could be used to treat arousal problems many drug companies changed their focus to testosterone treatments for low desire.

'The unnoticed shift in 2004 in FSD identity and promotion from female sexual arousal disorder to hypoactive sexual desire disorder is another hallmark moment in the FSD story, illustrating how the effort to match up some drug with FSD moved freely among symptoms and labels. By 2006, FSD has become a medical and media reality, despite the obvious ongoing difficulties in defining the condition and in getting a drug approved. Disease mongering has led to the successful "branding" of FSD, she said.

However, other clinicians insist that FSD is very much a reality for many women. Dr David Goldmeier runs one of the largest sexual function clinics in the UK and sees 150 women a year with FSD problems.

'If it is a problem for a woman – then it is a problem,' he says. 'The women I see are indeed profoundly affected. In my own sexual health unit, 20% of women who attended for a sexual infection screen felt they had significant sexual problems, and 60% of that 20% (i.e. 12%) wanted treatment for those problems. None of them had come to the clinic because of FSD (This study was not sponsored by the drug industry). Extrapolating over the whole of the UK that is a lot of women!

'I agree that many of these women may not actually have a disease. Some may be inconvenienced by their FSD, but most, I believe are stressed and pretty upset about their sexual problem. I do not medicalise FSD, rather I manage it by whatever means I feel appropriate. This can include reassurance, cognitive behaviour/sex therapy and medication where appropriate.'

Despite pioneering work by famous sexologists Kinsey and Masters and Johnson in the 1960s, what happens during female sexual arousal is still not completely understood. Accurate information about what happens is still lacking, although continuing research is breaking new ground.

There is even some confusion about basic physiology.

In 1998, Helen O'Connell, an Australian urologist, suggested that anatomy textbooks should be re-written following her discoveries about the size, positioning and functioning of the clitoris and its connection to the erectile tissue surrounding the urethra.

Advances in understanding are happening now because of more thorough investigation into physiological changes that occur before, during and after arousal and the use of scientific instruments to monitor these changes.

How is FSD determined?

'We had a very active sex life at the beginning and now I feel frustrated, cheated, I have decreased self-worth, I feel asexual, less feminine, and afraid that my partner will leave me. Will I be able to give him the feeling that I love him in an unrestricted and uninhibited way?'
– Julie, aged 40.

With no obvious erection stating 'yes, I am aroused' or 'no, I am not', women's sexual feelings have been considered far more subjective or controlled by their emotions. The direct parallel to erectile dysfunction, which affects one in 10 men is 'female arousal difficulty', one of the most common sexual problems for women.

Because we cannot see the complication as clearly as an erectile dysfunction, doctors might once have told women that their sexual problems were 'all in the head'. The added complication is that, unlike men with erectile dysfunction, women with arousal difficulty can still have intercourse even if they feel disinterested.

What happens during arousal?

Women experience swelling of erectile tissue during sexual arousal – they are not exactly erections as the tissues do not become rigid like an erect penis, but they certainly enlarge as the blood flows in. This flow of blood into the genitals provides medical researchers with an opportunity to learn about the female sexual response. There are now instruments which monitor the blood velocity and movement which create this tumescence and also very specific questionnaires which are helping to provide more of the answers.

WHAT IS SEXUAL AROUSAL ?

Researchers at the University of Amsterdam describe the female sexual response as a 'complicated bio-psychosocial' phenomenon. Psychologist Dr Ellen Laan says she believes arousal is triggered by a combination of external and internal stimulation (touch, smell, the sight of a loved one or sexual thoughts and fantasy) influenced by the central and the peripheral nervous system. This induces a need to participate in sex to satisfy the 'drive'.

Research in the United States suggests the vagus nerve which winds down through the body may be a 'sexual super highway' of the nervous system. The result of this double, inter-connected stimulation is a cascade of biochemical, hormonal and circulatory changes in the body which lead to the feeling associated with sexual arousal – the tingling, warmth, and nipple erection.

Sex hormones, or more specifically certain component parts, play a vital part in arousal and excitement. They act on sensory organs and can determine libido – the motivational force for sex. The clitoris, labia and even nipples are constructed of androgen-dependent tissues and, although

testosterone is generally considered to be a male hormone it is produced by the ovaries in women and is the 'fuel' which triggers the sex drive through its stimulating action upon androgen-dependent tissues As we age, levels of testosterone drop, and a shortage or imbalance may explain why some women do not experience sexual feelings (see chapter 8 – testosterone).

The next phase in this high-speed chain reaction is a flow of blood to the genitals triggered by chemical messengers and the nervous system, which responds within 20 seconds of an erotic thought. This leads to engorgement of the vagina, which triggers lubrication via the blood vessels, and the swelling of the clitoris and tissue around the urethra – the equivalent of a penis erecting.

Binding all these changes and influences are a woman's emotions, feelings or thoughts that can act as an override switch, turning off all the physical reactions as quickly as they were turned on. Previous sexual experiences can also play a part: some women need help to remove links between sexual response and negative feelings of guilt, anger or disgust. Cultural influences, parental attitudes, and one's own sense of self-esteem and self-worth can also play an important part.

1,410 men aged between 18 and 59. Their startling conclusion was that younger women are more likely to have problems with sexual desire and arousal than older women (apart from those who have trouble with lubrication leading to the problems of a dry vagina). A total of 43% of women reported significant problems with sexual desire, arousal or orgasm compared to 31% of men. Happiness, it suggested, is a key factor in a happy sex life. Emotional and physical satisfaction with the partner were of prime importance along with 'feelings of general happiness'.

The extent of the problem means there are potentially very many unhappy and sexually unfulfilled young and single women, most of whom are not aware they may be helped. It has been estimated that there are around 50 women of all ages in each GP's practice in the country who might need help for a sexual problem.

Alan Riley, the UK's first professor of sexual medicine at the University of Central Lancashire in Preston, conducted a pilot study among 100 women and found that 30% of women reported they had no sex drive whatsoever. He also discovered two peak ages for problems: the 30s and the 50s, confirming the US finding.

A survey at one of the country's specialist clinics for female sexual dysfunction – the Jane Waddington Clinic at St Mary's Hospital London – found that 60% of the women interviewed had experienced some sort of sexual problem – 22% reported problems with orgasm and 25% with vaginismus (a spasm of the vaginal muscles which blocks the entrance to the vagina). Around two-thirds said they would like to have treatment, one-third said they did not.

The first survey[2] of the extent and nature of sexual problems in the UK has shown how common they are – affecting 43% of women – that is four women in every 10. Only a small number had had help for their problem – although a large number wanted help. The survey was carried out in four GP practices in England among 789 men and 979 women and concluded:

- one-third of the respondents had not had sex in the previous three months
- 41% of women reported having one or more sexual problems during the previous three months
- the most common female problems were: vaginal dryness and orgasm difficulties
- sexual intercourse was never or rarely a pleasant experience for 110 of the women

YOUNG AND OLD

Unmarried women are 1.5 times as likely to have sexual problems involving orgasm and sexual anxiety than married women. A US report suggests that women in stable relationships and long-term marriages enjoy their sex lives better than young women who may have a high incidence of 'partner turnover'.

- 68% reported having some sort of sexual problem at some time previously
- but only 4% of women had received help

The problem is widespread: yet very little is being done for affected women – partly because few seek help many women are not sure where to go. Apart from the GP, the genito-urinary clinic, or sexual and marital therapists who take a mainly psychological approach, there are very few clinics offering specific sexual help for women from a medical perspective although, since this book was first published more have sprung up. Little attention is paid to the fact that women may often also feel happier talking to another woman about these problems.

Dr Frances Quirk conducted the world's first study into the impact of sex problems on women's quality of life for Pfizer. During her two years of research, Dr Quirk tapped into a 'great well of unhappiness' being endured by women with sex problems; many of whom felt their condition was not being adequately dealt with or even properly understood by either their partner or their doctor. Her findings are leading to a greater understanding of women's sexual dysfunction and, along with work being conducted in the US and elsewhere, may contribute to greater understanding and definition of sexual disorders for doctors.

She conducted or supervised 82 face-to-face detailed and often highly-emotional interviews with women. Some had kept their problems and feelings bottled up for a long time and wept openly about the poor state of their sex lives, which was directly affecting them and their close relationships, as well as creating feelings of insecurity about their partners.

Many women felt disempowered, and were deeply hurt that their self-worth and self-esteem seemed to be irreparably damaged. Others were worried that their husbands would leave them. From these interviews, Dr Quirk developed a questionnaire which was randomly sent out to 1,160 women. More than 72% replied and of those, 400 said they had recently suffered or were suffering one of six sexual problems listed in the questionnaire.

Dr Quirk was particularly keen to find out about difficulties with sexual arousal and loss of sexual interest because these are described by women as the major problems in almost every sexual health survey in the UK or USA. Her work confirmed this:

- 50% of women who said they had sexual problems said they suffered or had suffered a recent 'lack of interest' in sex
- 30% said they took a long time to become aroused
- a further 26% said they had difficulty becoming aroused.

Other complaints were:
- lack of lubrication (24%)
- pain or discomfort having sex (35%)
- difficulty achieving orgasm (28%)

Many women had several of these problems.

The sexual quality of life survey focused on the impact of the social, physical, emotional and psychological consequences of sexual problems and concluded that large numbers of women simply do not have satisfactory sex lives. Many women who have arousal or loss of interest problems have a very poor quality of life sexually.
The survey revealed that

- a quarter of women with sexual arousal problems do not find their sexual life an enjoyable part of their life overall
- nearly 30% are not satisfied with the frequency of sex
- nearly 1 in 5 of the women had lost all pleasure in sex.
- a third of the women worried about the future of their sex lives

As this was a random survey, the women who returned their questionnaires were ordinary women in the UK – a cross-section, and, because of this, these results undoubtedly reflect what is happening in the lives of any given group of 1,000 women in the UK. Of the women who responded, 80% had a partner, 96% had had a relationship in the past six months and 84% had children.

In other words, the sex lives of many women in this country seem to be in a shocking state – yet there are few clinics or clinicians available to help. Indeed many women do not think they can be helped. Not surprisingly, the survey also revealed that more than 40% of women with sexual problems avoid having sex and worry about their future sex lives.

An interesting insight into women's understanding of sexual problems was shown by the 5 to 10% of women who said they have never had a sexual problem.

How the research was conducted

In order to find out how sex problems affect women's lives, Dr Quirk devised an easy-to-understand questionnaire, choosing words women would use themselves to describe their sexual problems.

She initially interviewed 82 women in six different countries – 22 of whom had sought help for sexual problems although the interviews also disclosed that a further 12 had one or more of the key sexual problems (such as a loss of arousal, lack of interest, problems with attaining orgasm, lubrication difficulty or pain on intercourse) although they had not sought help. It was through these one-to-one interviews that she tapped deep into the heart of the problem and faced, for the first time, the enormity of the problem and the unhappiness a life without sex can mean. It has an impact on the women, and their families: possibly even the family structure.

Many women worried their husbands would leave them because of their problem – a lack of interest in sex, or an inability to feel sexually aroused.

Why women complain in such large numbers about their loss of interest in partners, or 'going off sex' is a major focus of the current work and research on sexual dysfunctions in women. But it still remains something of a medical mystery – although more answers to this will come as scientists and clinicians focus on the problem.

However, there is wider recognition and acceptance of the fact that a large proportion of women suffer from a sexual dysfunction at some stage in their lives. This recognition has only just started to filter down to doctors, and, most importantly affected women themselves.

The next step will be finding solutions. Medication is unlikely to be the total solution to the problems: there also must be a place for sex therapy, and relationship counselling – and sometimes these will be more appropriate.

Dr Quirk began her quest by finding out what women thought about sexual arousal and arousal problems. 'I wanted to know what they deemed sexual arousal to be and what were women's signals for becoming sexually aroused. I wanted to know about the normal sexual response in women and what women consider sexual arousal to mean, before moving on to find out about the impact of female sexual dysfunction on women's sexual quality of life. I was interested in how women described these signals and what language they used.'

She says: 'Sexual interest and arousal for a man are not necessarily perceived or understood in the same way as sexual interest and arousal for a woman. There are many interlinking factors for women. For women, sexual arousal may be far more complex, and both sexual interest and arousal are more deeply inter-related than has been previously understood.

'One of the things which became clear is that the signals women interpret as relating to arousal are both emotional and psychological. They might mention that arousal means being more lubricated, they are more sensitive to touch, but they also mention that they felt much closer to their partner and the emotional side which was just as important as the physical side in terms of feeling aroused.'

What the result of the research will mean

Dr Quirk's work is part of a move towards a greater understanding of female sexual response and female sexual dysfunction. It will lead to new clinical definitions and possible future treatments.

Female sexual dysfunctions are currently classified as discrete disorders in one of the phases of the sexual response cycle – desire, arousal, orgasm,– or pain related to sexual activity. The problems have led to the terms – *disorders of*

- Sexual drive
- Arousal
- Orgasm
- Pain

These are the descriptions used in the Diagnostics and Statistical Manual (DSMIV), a psychiatric diagnostic manual used by clinicians. But researchers say that because the symptoms often overlap, this diagnostic tool is outdated. It was developed to help classify problems for psychiatric disorders but lacks objectivity for sexual disorders which may have a biological influence.

Dr Quirk's work in the late 1990s talking to real women with real problems revealed how much more inter-related the phases are and how each phase is more complex than previously recognised.

She has helped to create the Sexual Function Questionnaire (reproduced on page 34) which can be used to help ascertain whether women have FSD or not and detect any change in their sexual function, and the Sexual Quality of Life Questionnaire which assesses the impact of sexual problems on a woman's quality of life.

Dr Quirk discovered that the problems women faced with their sexuality knew no national boundaries – there were no cultural differences separating the women. Those who felt living without joyful sex was a deep loss, she says, were all desperately seeking a solution to what, until now, has been their 'secret' and hidden problem, largely misunderstood not only by doctors but also their partners.

New definitions for female sexual dysfunctions created by a panel, sponsored by the American Foundation for Urologic Disease (AFUD), in 2000 reflect recent increases in understanding[3].

This international panel agreed that the four main titles for sexual disorders should remain – desire, arousal, orgasm and pain (dyspareunia) – but that some changes to the definitions of each disorder were timely.

The definition of desire disorder now takes account of personal distress in relation to any desire problem, and deficiency in sexual thoughts, desire for or receptivity to sexual activity. The definition for arousal disorder also includes the element of 'personal distress' as well as elaborating on how difficulty with arousal might be experienced by including lack of subjective excitement, genital and other 'somatic' responses.

Researchers have also recently identified three separate categories within FSAD, which take into account the context in which a woman experiences arousal difficulties, for example if she is in a destructive relationship or is living in poverty. These are explained on page 30. A report published in the *Journal of Sex & Marriage Therapy* in 2005 argues that re-classification of FSAD could help to improve diagnostic accuracy, leading to more successful treatment[4].

Any future measurements of female sexual dysfunction will inevitably have to take into account the thoughts and emotions a woman experiences when she is having problems with sex.

Summary
It is easy to diagnose erectile dysfunction in a man but how do women recognise the symptoms of female arousal disorders?

When it comes to sex do you:

- have internal physical reactions such as warmth, tingling and genital sensations when you are sexually stimulated?
- experience increase in vaginal lubrication (wetness) in response to sexual stimulation?
- feel 'excited' or 'turned on' in response to sexual stimulation?
- want sexual activity to continue once it has started?

If the answer is 'no' to all these questions and this has been part of a consistent pattern over a reasonable period of time (e.g. 6 months) and it distresses you, then you may be experiencing an arousal disorder.

The questionnaire at the end of this chapter will help to determine what profile of sexual function you have currently. A high level of sexual symptoms may indicate that you have a sexual problem or may simply reflect your current circumstances.

A diagnosis of a sexual disorder could only be made with additional information; such as whether any relationship issues exist and whether the sexual symptoms reported have been consistent over a period of time and cause you distress.

Using a questionnaire defining sexual dysfunction not only helps researchers to understand the extent of the problem – and how women view it – but can also be used to determine how successful new therapies might be. FSD is a global expression covering a wide range of sexual problems affecting women. FSD is not straightforward. But there are various disorders, which are usually explored by clinicians with an interest in the problem although an affected woman may suffer from one or a combination of these conditions.

Lack of sexual drive

It is estimated that 30% of women with sexual dysfunction problems have no sex drive – the biological force which makes someone seek out or accept sex. Affected women have no need for sex (unless they want to have a baby). A zero sex drive is most likely to have a biological, or physical, explanation. This is a recent finding and it is pushing forward the research into treatments and causes.

SYMPTOMS

- no desire to initiate sex .
- no desire to participate in sex unless trying for a baby but may seek comfort from cuddling alone without penetration
- no receptivity to sexual advances or activity

POSSIBLE PHYSICAL CAUSES

- low testosterone levels
- high blood pressure
- thyroid disease

- high prolactin levels (the hormone which circulates during breast feeding)
- alcohol or drug problems
- diabetes

TESTS
- hormone levels checked
- thyroid function monitored
- biofeedback to monitor blood flow

TREATMENTS
- use of hormonal creams
- treatment for an underlying condition, such as thyroid problems or diabetes
- oxytocin – researchers are looking at whether it may be a useful pro-sexual drug

Lack of sexual desire or ISD (inhibited sexual desire)

The number of women with reduced sexual desire has increased substantially over the past 20 years, according to Prof. Riley of the University of Lancashire. It is the most frequent complaint among women attending sex therapy clinics, affecting 80% of women who seek help.

Women who lose their desire may not have lost their ability to become aroused and may be quite capable of having good sex with orgasm. They may 'learn' to lose interest in sex because of pain, a bad experience or something off-putting – it could as simple as a partner having dirty fingernails.

Women who lose their sexual desire may still want to be loved and held by their partners but may not want penetration. However, this signal can be wrongly misinterpreted by the partner as a desire for sex, leading to a build-up of hostility and then guilt. Loss of sexual desire can be confused with loss of drive: tests can show a woman that she is responding in the right way physically and help her to recognise those feelings.

SYMPTOMS
- loss of sexual spark
- little desire to initiate sex although if stimulated properly can still achieve orgasm
- aversion to sexual overtures
- distress or emotional upset

POSSIBLE CAUSES
- extreme tiredness
- depression or use of certain anti-depressants
- androgen deficiency (after hysterectomy, removal of ovaries, or chemotherapy for cancer)

- alcohol or drug abuse
- urological, obstetric or gynaecological complications which cause pain when having sex, such as vaginismus and vestibulitis
- a psychological block because of a previous bad experience or parental influence
- obesity and loss of self-esteem
- general unhappiness in relationships or with partner
- stress or anxiety with work or home
- unresolved sexual orientation
- previous traumatic sexual experience
- the contraceptive pill can sometimes inhibit desire

TESTS
- hormone levels checked
- assessment of anti-depressant drugs
- gynaecological check-up
- review of contraception

TREATMENTS
- psycho-sexual counselling
- testosterone treatment
- a change in type and hormonal content of the birth control pill
- alcohol or drugs counselling
- weight loss plan
- stimulation of the sympathetic nervous system – through exercise or 'excitement' which raises blood pressure and heart rate

Lack of sexual arousal or FSAD (female sexual arousal disorder)

Female sexual arousal disorder can occur on its own, or in combination with either of the other two problems. It is very likely to have a physical cause and research has defined two problems – vascular and clitoral erectile insufficiency syndrome: which means that arterial disease might influence blood flow and the subsequent required engorgement of clitoral, vaginal and urethral tissues.

Like a man with erectile dysfunction, a woman's sexual responses can sometimes fail because of a physical problem in the complex sexual circuitry. During normal arousal a woman's clitoris and the tissues surrounding the vaginal opening become engorged with blood rather like a penis does. The clitoris has the same nerve endings as a penis, and enlarges during arousal. At the same time the vagina elongates to receive the penis.

Furthermore, physiologists now believe that in normal arousal the erectile tissues around the urethra expand to produce pleasurable sensations. It is perhaps not surprising: both male and female genitals develop from the same sort of fetal tissue (anlagen, a German word meaning the same) which in maturity reacts in a similar way to sexual stimulation.

In 2004, Basson *et al* identified three separate categories of FSAD [5]. These are:

PHYSICAL OR GENITAL SEXUAL AROUSAL DISORDER:
Physical sexual arousal is absent or reduced. Sexual stimulation results in only minimal clitoral swelling or vaginal lubrication and sexual sensations from sexually caressing the genitals, breasts and other areas are reduced. Subjective sexual excitement and sexual pleasure still occur, typically from non-genital stimulation.

PSYCHOLOGICAL SEXUAL AROUSAL DISORDER:
Subjective sexual pleasure from any type of sexual stimulation is absent or greatly diminished, although vaginal lubrication or other signs of physical response still occur.

COMBINED PHYSICAL AND SEXUAL AROUSAL DISORDER:
Little or no subjective sexual excitement or feelings of sexual pleasure from any type of sexual stimulation as well as little or no physical sexual arousal.

SYMPTOMS
- an inability to lubricate – leading to vaginal dryness – affecting mostly older women
- no erotic sensations or feelings of heightened sexual excitement
- reduced or absent orgasm (anorgasmia)
- pain with intercourse
- diminished vaginal sensation

POSSIBLE CAUSES
- physiological complication such as an impairment of the blood flow to the clitoris or vagina, or nerve damage around the urethra, vagina, or clitoris
- lack of adequate stimulation from partner/lack of ability to arouse partner
- arterial or vascular disease
- chronic disease such as epilepsy, kidney failure
- multiple sclerosis
- hormonal changes at the menopause
- pelvic injury damaging the arteries leading to the vagina and clitoris. restricting the blood flow

TESTS
- Doppler imaging to monitor blood changes in the genitalia

- blood tests for chronic illness
- hormonal checks
- nerve assessment treatments
- combined HRT and methyl testosterone (still considered controversial by some doctors)
- change in diet
- vitamin, mineral or herbal supplements
- improved happiness through relaxation and exercise
- alternative therapies
- change in sexual techniques and new sexual stimulation
- topical vaginal oestrogens for peri- and post-menopausal women
- artificial lubricants, such as KY-jelly

Painful sex

This can be long or short term and caused by a different vulval disorders. There may also be a psychological cause for pain that needs resolving (*see chapter six: painful sex*).

Female orgasmic disorder (FOD)

Some women complain of not being able to achieve orgasm even though they feel sexually aroused and responsive. This is a common problem. The problem for clinicians is establishing what is 'normal' — female orgasmic ability varies hugely. Some women can become orgasmic with nipple stimulation and fantasy; some need long periods of clitoral stimulation; others are never able to achieve orgasm. There is probably a significant psychological element in orgasm disorders (*see chapter four — sex and the mind*).

Factors needed for good sex

Physical

- genital response
- no pain
- engorgement through blood flow to the vagina, clitoris and labia
- correct levels of testosterone, the hormone which affects the sex drive
- healthy, working sensory nerves to provide and send the pleasurable feelings to the brain via spinal cord
- lubrication to aid penetration — otherwise it will be painful. The blood flow to the vagina facilitates lubrication.

Psychological or emotional

- psychological empathy, 'desire' or emotional contact with partner
- the 'drive' or need to participate in sex with a partner

- the need to feel comfortable with what is happening, free of anxiety, anger and distraction.
- an ability to let go and enjoy the experience without 'sex guilt'

IF THESE BASICS ARE NOT IN PLACE THE OUTCOME IS:

- dry vagina and pain
- inadequate engorgement of the labia, making vaginal opening difficult
- if the uterus is not elevated during intercourse, the cervix tends to stay fixed in one place, and this coupled with poor vaginal engorgement will lead to painful buffeting
- reduced genital sensation
- no response to sexual stimulus
- no desire to want to make love

What women really, really want

Researchers at the Robert Wood Johnson Medical School in New Jersey, USA make the pertinent point that doctors should consider what women really want from sex. For many women sexual satisfaction includes affection, communication with their partner, and sensual touching. They say that attraction, passion, trust and intimacy are more significant than their genital response. Some women find that specific problems can put them off sex, and cause them to lose their desire for sex. These specific problems – such as painful sex – are explored in later chapters.

References

[1]Laumann, E. O., Glasser, D. B., Nicolosi, A., Brock, G., Moreira, E., Gingell, C. The Impact of Biological Aging Effects on the reporting of Sexual Dysfunctions in Women aged 40-80 years: Results of an international survey. Presented at the Society for the Study of Women's Sexual Health, Vancouver, October 2002.

[2]Dunn, K .M., Croft, P. R., Hackett, G. I. Sexual problems: a study of the prevalence and need for health care in the general population. *Family Practice* 1998. **15**: 519-24.

[3]Basson, R. *et al*. Report of the International Consensus Development Conference on Female Sexual Dysfunction: Definitions and Classification. *The Journal of Urology* 2000. **163**: 888-893.

[4]Althof, S. *et al*. Outcome Measurement in Female Sexual Dysfunction Clinical Trials: Review and Recommendations. *Journal of Sex & Marital Therapy* 2005. **31**:153–166, 2005.

[5]Basson, R. *et al*. Definitions of women's sexual dysfunction reconsidered: Advocating expansion and revision. *Journal of Psychosomatic Obstetrics and Gynecology* 2004. **24**: 221–229.

female sexual function questionnaire

These questions ask about a sensitive topic, your sexual activity and your sexual life with your partner. We have defined 'sexual activity' as activity which may result in sexual stimulation or sexual pleasure. Sexual activity may not always involve a partner. We have defined 'sexual life' as both physical sexual activities and the emotional sexual relationship that you have with your partner. The questionnaire can only be completed (to be scored) if some sexual activity has taken place over the last month. If the questions don't apply to you, move on to the next one. Please answer the questions as honestly and candidly as you can and refer to the side panels for an explanation of the scoring system.

SFQ SCORING SYSTEM

Individual Items
The SFQ contains 33 items and each item has between 5 or 7 possible answers.

Items **1-6, 14, 16, 20-21, 23-28** and **32-33** are scored 1-5 (in **ascending** order) e.g. question **1.** Over the last four weeks, how often have you had pleasurable thoughts and feelings about sexual activity?

Not at all	**(1)**
Rarely	**(2)**
Sometimes	**(3)**
Often	**(4)**
Very often	**(5)**

Section 1 : Sexual Activity

These questions ask about your sexual activity over the last four weeks. Please answer every question by marking one box with a cross. If you are unsure about how to answer, please give the best answer you can. In answering these questions the following definition of 'sexual activity' applies:

- Sexual activity – includes any activity which may result in sexual stimulation or sexual pleasure e.g. intercourse, caressing, foreplay, masturbation (i.e. self-masturbation or your partner masturbating you) and oral sex (i.e., your partner giving you oral sex).

1. Over the last four weeks, how often have you had pleasurable thoughts and feelings about sexual activity?
Please cross one box only
- ❏ Not at all
- ❏ Rarely
- ❏ Sometimes
- ❏ Often
- ❏ Very often

2. Over the last four weeks, how often have you wanted to be sensually touched and caressed by your partner?
Please cross one box only
- ❏ Not at all
- ❏ Rarely
- ❏ Sometimes
- ❏ Often
- ❏ Very often

3. Over the last four weeks, how often have you wanted to take part in sexual activity?
Please cross one box only
- ❏ Not at all
- ❏ Rarely
- ❏ Sometimes
- ❏ Often
- ❏ Very often

4. Over the last four weeks, how often have you initiated sexual activity with your partner?
Please cross one box only
- ❏ Not at all
- ❏ Rarely
- ❏ Sometimes
- ❏ Often
- ❏ Very often

5. Over the last four weeks, how often have you been sensually touched and caressed by your partner?
Please cross one box only
- ❏ Not at all
- ❏ Rarely
- ❏ Sometimes
- ❏ Often
- ❏ Very often

6. Over the last four weeks, in general, how enjoyable has it been to be sensually touched and caressed by your partner?
Please cross one box only
- ❏ Not enjoyable
- ❏ Slightly enjoyable
- ❏ Moderately enjoyable

- ❏ Very enjoyable
- ❏ Extremely enjoyable

7. Over the last four weeks, how often did you have a feeling of 'warmth' in your vagina/genital area when you took part in sexual activity?
Please cross one box only
- ❏ Not at all
- ❏ Sometimes
- ❏ Often
- ❏ Very often
- ❏ Every time

8. Over the last four weeks, in general, how much 'warmth' did you feel in your vagina/genital area when you took part in sexual activity?
Please cross one box only
- ❏ None
- ❏ Slightly 'warm'
- ❏ Moderately 'warm'
- ❏ Very 'warm'
- ❏ Extremely 'warm'

9. Over the last four weeks, how often did you have a sensation of 'pulsating' ('tingling') in your vagina/genital area when you took part in sexual activity?
Please cross one box only
- ❏ Not at all
- ❏ Sometimes
- ❏ Often
- ❏ Very often
- ❏ Every time

Items **15** and **19** are scored 0-6 (in **ascending** order)

Items **17-18**, **29**, **30** and **31** are scored 5-1 (in **descending** order)

Not at all	**(5)**
Slightly	**(4)**
Moderately	**(3)**
Very	**(2)**
Extremely	**(1)**

Item **22** is scored from 5-1 in **descending** order

10. Over the last four weeks, in general, how much 'pulsating' ('tingling') in your vagina/genital area did you notice when you took part in sexual activity?
Please cross one box only
❑ No sensation
❑ A mild sensation
❑ A moderate sensation
❑ A strong sensation
❑ A very strong sensation

11. Over the last four weeks, how often did you notice vaginal wetness/lubrication when you took part in sexual activity?
Please cross one box only
❑ Not at all
❑ Sometimes
❑ Often
❑ Very often
❑ Every time

12. Over the last four weeks, in general, how much vaginal wetness/lubrication did you notice when you took part in sexual activity?
Please cross one box only
❑ No wetness/lubrication
❑ Slightly wet/lubricated
❑ Moderately wet/lubricated
❑ Very wet/lubricated
❑ Extremely wet/lubricated

13. Over the last four weeks, how often did you have feelings of emotional sexual arousal when you took part in sexual activity? (e.g. feeling

excited, feeling 'turned on', wanting sexual activity to continue)
Please cross one box only
❑ Not at all
❑ Sometimes
❑ Often
❑ Very often
❑ Every time

14. Over the last four weeks, how much emotional sexual arousal did you notice when you took part in sexual activity? (e.g. feeling excited, feeling 'turned on', wanting sexual activity to continue)
Please cross one box only
❑ None
❑ Slightly aroused
❑ Moderately aroused
❑ Very aroused
❑ Extremely aroused

15. Over the last four weeks, how often did you take part in sexual activity with penetration (e.g. vaginal penetration and intercourse)?
Please cross one box only
❑ I did not take part in sexual activity
❑ Once/twice
❑ 3-4 times
❑ 5-8 times
❑ 9-12 times
❑ 13-16 times
❑ 16 times

16. Over the last four weeks, in general, how much did you enjoy penetration and intercourse?
Please cross one box only
❏ Not enjoyable
❏ Slightly enjoyable
❏ Moderately enjoyable
❏ Very enjoyable
❏ Extremely enjoyable

17. Over the last four weeks, how often did you experience pain in your vagina/genital area during or after sexual activity (e.g. penetration, intercourse)?
Please cross one box only
❏ Not at all
❏ Sometimes
❏ Often
❏ Very often
❏ Every time

18. Over the last four weeks, in general, how much pain did you experience in your vagina/genital area during or after sexual activity (e.g. penetration, intercourse)?
Please cross one box only
❏ No pain
❏ Slightly painful
❏ Moderately painful
❏ Very painful
❏ Extremely painful

19. Over the last four weeks, how often did you take part in sexual activity without penetration (e.g. masturbation, oral sex)?
Please cross one box only
❏ I did not take part in sexual activity without penetration
❏ Once/twice
❏ 3-4 times
❏ 5-8 times
❏ 9-12 times
❏ 13-16 times
❏ 16 times

20. Over the last four weeks, in general, how much did you enjoy sexual activity without penetration (e.g. masturbation, oral sex)?
Please cross one box only
❏ No enjoyment
❏ Slightly enjoyable
❏ Moderately enjoyable
❏ Very enjoyable
❏ Extremely enjoyable

21. Over the last four weeks, how often did you feel emotionally close to your partner when you took part in sexual activity?
Please cross one box only
❏ Not at all
❏ Sometimes
❏ Often
❏ Very often
❏ Every time

22. Over the last four weeks, how often have you been worried or anxious about pain during sexual activity?
Please cross one box only

☐ Not at all
☐ Sometimes
☐ Often
☐ Very often
☐ Every time

23. Over the last four weeks, did you feel good about yourself when you were sexually active?
Please cross one box only
☐ Not at all
☐ Slightly
☐ Moderately
☐ Very
☐ Extremely

24. Over the last four weeks, how often did you have an orgasm when you took part in sexual activity (may be with or without a partner)?
Please cross one box only
☐ Not at all
☐ Sometimes
☐ Often
☐ Very often
☐ Every time

25. Over the last four weeks, in general, how pleasurable were the orgasms that you had?

Please cross one box only
☐ I did not have any orgasms
☐ Not pleasurable
☐ Slightly pleasurable
☐ Moderately pleasurable
☐ Very pleasurable
☐ Extremely pleasurable

26. Over the last four weeks, in general, how easy was it for you to reach orgasm?
Please cross one box only
☐ Very difficult
☐ Quite difficult
☐ Neither easy or difficult
☐ Quite easy
☐ Very easy
☐ I did not have any orgasms

27. Over the last four weeks, how confident have you felt about yourself as a sexual partner?
Please cross one box only
☐ Not at all
☐ Slightly
☐ Moderately
☐ Very
☐ Extremely

Section 2 : Sexual Life

These questions ask about your sexual life over the last four weeks. Please answer every question by marking one box with a cross. If you are unsure about how to answer, please give the best answer you can. The following questions ask about both positive and negative feelings regarding your sexual life. In answering these questions the following definition of 'sexual life' applies:

- **Sexual life** – both the physical sexual activities and the emotional sexual relationship that you have with your partner.

28. Thinking about your sexual life over the last four weeks, how often did you look forward to sexual activity?
Please cross one box only
- ☐ Not at all
- ☐ Rarely
- ☐ Sometimes
- ☐ Often
- ☐ Very often

29. Thinking about your sexual life over the last four weeks, did you feel disappointed with your sexual response (e.g. ability to become aroused, lubrication)?
Please cross one box only
- ☐ Not at all
- ☐ Slightly
- ☐ Moderately
- ☐ Very
- ☐ Extremely

30. Thinking about the last 4 weeks, how much did you worry that your partner may look for another sexual relationship because of problems with your sexual life?
Please cross one box only

- ☐ Not at all
- ☐ Slightly
- ☐ Moderately
- ☐ Very
- ☐ Extremely

31. Thinking about the last four weeks, how much did you worry about your partner's negative feelings about your sexual life (e.g. partner feeling angry, hurt, rejected)?
Please cross one box only
- ☐ Not at all
- ☐ Slightly
- ☐ Moderately
- ☐ Very
- ☐ Extremely

32. Over the last four weeks, taking the whole of your sexual life into account, how satisfied have you been?
Please cross one box only
- ☐ Not satisfied
- ☐ Slightly satisfied
- ☐ Moderately satisfied
- ☐ Very satisfied
- ☐ Extremely satisfied

33. In general, how important is being able to have an enjoyable sexual life to you?

Please cross one box only
☐ Not at all
☐ Slightly
☐ Moderately
☐ Very
☐ Extremely **(5)**

Total Score

Your total score is reached by adding up the scores for the individual questions. The total score range is 30-167. A higher score indicates better sexual function. This questionnaire will help you to identify if you have a particular problem – see the headings listed below in the left hand column.

Domain	Score range indicating high probability of FSD	Score range indicating borderline sexual function	Score range indicating high probability of normal sexual function
Desire (Qs 1-4, 15, 28)	5-16	17-22	23-31
Arousal (S) (Qs 7-10)	4-10	11-13	14-20
Arousal (L) (Qs 11-12)	2-5	6-7	8-10
Orgasm (Qs 24-26)	3-8	9-11	12-15
Pain (Qs 17, 18, 22)	2-8	9-11	12-15
Enjoyment (Qs 6, 16, 20, 21, 23, 27)	6-16	17-22	23-30

High probability of FSD only if symptoms present for 6 months, no other issues and personal distress. Arousal (S) is Arousal sensation. Arousal (L) is Arousal lubrication.

3

sex and physiology

'If I met someone who said that I could regain my sexual feelings, I would do almost anything – I'd say, let's go for it. But as time goes by I've rationalised my feelings – this is where I am now,'
Martine, aged in her 60s, suffering from an inability to become sexually aroused.

Scientists are still pushing forward frontiers of understanding about female physiology in relation to sex and sexual responses. One woman researcher working in the field summed up the general lack of knowledge as 'woefully horrendous'.

Despite greater openness about sexuality today many women have very little understanding of their own bodies or exactly what happens during sexual arousal. This chapter aims to explain a little more about the cascade of physical responses and also how they are linked to our emotions and psychological responses.

To understand the disorders of female sexual dysfunction it helps to understand what happens during the normal response. Although research is on-going and parts of the jigsaw puzzle still falling into place, Helen O'Connell, based at the Royal Melbourne Hospital in Australia, says that 'more systematic physiological studies are required'. Drug companies currently employ some of the most eminent doctors and scientists working in sexual medicine to test the effectiveness of a small range of drugs for women and to find out more about the physiology of females.

Dr Mitra Boolell, former clinical leader at Pfizer, the company that first started looking at new therapies for FSD in 1996, says: 'It was clear to us right from the start how little people understood FSD.

'FSD is very common but it is amazing how under-recognised it is.' In any group of

100 women there are likely to be between 20 and 27 who have trouble lubricating and have arousal difficulties alone. It cuts across the age band and is four times as prevalent as ED in men.' He adds that the under-recognition of the problem by doctors is partly historical. 'As a doctor myself, the amount of training we got in sexual health I could summarise in half an hour.'

Taking a different view are psychologists trying to determine the importance of the mind and the brain in the arousal process and a woman's ability to 'let go' or lose control during sex which they believe is equally as important as the mechanical aspects. This is explored more in *chapter four: sex and the mind*.

Just a decade or so ago, erectile dysfunction in men was thought to be mainly psychological except in the obvious cases of paralysis and injury. But now it is acknowledged that between 70 and 90 per cent of cases have physical causes. This discovery has launched a new industry: medication, which, it is estimated, can help 70% of affected men. But will it do the same for women? A few women with certain problems connected with blood flow to and engorgement of the genitals may be helped, particularly if the drugs are given in conjunction with psychotherapy. At present most of the research is focused on postmenopausal women or those who have had hysterectomies.

The key elements of sexual arousal

Dr Roy Levin is a physiologist at Sheffield University and has been studying the female sexual response for 30 years. He is now considered the 'grandfather' of this field of research, but admits that three decades ago 'no-one was interested'.

One of his findings published in the *Archives of Sexual Behavior*[1] may have repercussions for doctors working with infertile couples. Changes caused by sexual arousal have implications for both the enjoyment of sex and successful reproduction, he says.

When a woman is aroused the vagina balloons – creating a 'holding place' for sperm, delaying its transport to the fallopian tubes, allowing it to 'de-coagulate' and thereby possibly increasing the chances of fertilisation. In a non-aroused woman, sperm travels to the fallopian tubes much more quickly and this speed may affect both its quality and viability.

All this, he says, could have implications for couples experiencing fertility problems. Dr Levin's work is considered to be some of the

IN THE BEGINNING ...

In the womb we are all alike for the first six to eight weeks. The Y-chromosome makes a testis occur from the indifferent gonad (the ovotestis). The ovotestis is internal waiting to become an ovary or a testis and the tubercle is external, a superficial structure mainly waiting to become a penis/scrotum or clitoris. In boys the fetal testis then secretes testosterone which acts locally to support and differentiate the Wolffian ducts which make the male 'plumbing',

most detailed of its kind and is a reference point for much of the new wave of research, which is why he is in demand as a speaker at international conferences.

In one key work[2] he says: 'Human sexual desire is complex and is not a single entity, it can change during the sexual scenario experienced by a person. Four practically serial sub-categories of sexual desire usually occur during an encounter – wanting sexual activity/arousal to occur; wanting to create sexual arousal in another person; wanting intercourse to happen; and wanting orgasm to occur. It is possible to have sexual desire without sexual arousal and sexual arousal without desire.'

Dr Levin suggests that some women may suffer sexually because they are simply not being stimulated effectively by their partners due to:
- a lack of awareness (by both partners) of the female genital anatomy
- what happens during arousal
- where the important sexually arousable zones are positioned

Although people are aware of the clitoris and the G-spot – or more accurately the G-area – there is very little published information on other parts of the genitalia which can be stimulated erotically. Most women regard their genitals as rather mysterious and take the 'would prefer not to know' attitude, Dr Levin believes. 'Most women have never seen their genitals – most women hate the idea.' But, he says if women and men understood more about what happens, this alone might dramatically improve their sex lives. Also, he points out, there is individual variation to take into account. 'You get a whole range of behaviours and a whole range of anatomical variations – for example labia are as individual as noses and the sensitivity of them will vary.'

In published papers, Dr Levin has listed several 'arousable' areas in the female genitalia. Research suggests that these areas may be inter-connected which might explain why some Sudanese women who have clitorectomies say that later they are still able to achieve orgasm.

The elements involved in physical arousal
STIMULATION POINTS FOR GOOD SEX

INTERNALLY
- the G-spot or area
- the urethra

and via, the blood, to the external genital tubercle which develops into the penis/scrotum. The fetal testis also makes a chemical which inhibits the development of the so-called Mullerian duct which develops into the female genitals. In boys, the genital tubercle grows into the penis which grows outwards. The scrotal and urethral folds fuse together to form the scrotum. In girls, the genital tubercle becomes the clitoris which, it is now known, grows inwards and wraps around the urethra. The tissue that becomes the scrotum in boys

- Halban's fascia*
- the cervix
- the muscles around the vagina

positioned in the space between the bladder and the top wall of the vagina, this area is filled with collagen, elastin and muscle fibre and has a rich blood and nerve supply. Some medical researchers believe this to be the female equivalent of the corpus spongiosum *in men. On sexual stimulation this layer engorges with blood.*

EXTERNALLY

- the clitoris
- the labia
- P-spot or area

THE PHYSIOLOGICAL RESPONSE TO SEXUAL AROUSAL

- increased pulse and heart rate
- increased skin temperature
- lubrication of the vagina
- pink flush on the chest
- breast enlargement and nipple erection
- swelling of labia and clitoris
- vaginal expansion and uterine and cervical elevation

The P-spot or area

It was always thought that the clitoral shaft and glans in the female was equivalent to the penile shaft and glans because it develops from a common tissue in the fetus.

However, in 1987 it was argued that the clitoris in women was not a direct equivalent with the penis in men. It was pointed out that in men the urethra courses through the penile glans while this was not the case for the clitoris.

A researcher, E. Sevely, argued that the real equivalent in women was an area of mucous membrane surrounding the urethral opening and stretching from just below the clitoris to the top of the vaginal opening. This area was only given an anatomical name in 1989 by Sevely who called it the 'female glans'.

However Dr Levin believes a better name for this area is the periurethral glans which I have termed, colloquially, the P-area or the P-spot. He investigated whether this area is highly sensitive to erotic stimulation and published his results in 1991. In this work, Dr Levin

---

becomes the inner and outer labial folds.

In men and women there are two types of erectile tissue which engorge upon sexual stimulation. The *corpus cavernosa* is the tissue, which provides the erection in men and the swelling of the clitoris in women. The *corpus spongiosum* surrounds the urethra in men and is 'sponge-like'. In women this type of tissue surrounds the vaginal bulbs, glans of the clitoris and sit under the periurethral area.

Section through female pelvic region

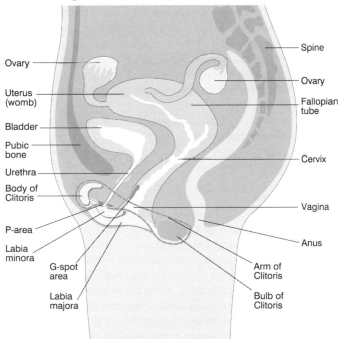

Spine
Ovary
Ovary
Uterus (womb)
Fallopian tube
Bladder
Pubic bone
Cervix
Urethra
Body of Clitoris
Vagina
P-area
Anus
Labia minora
G-spot area
Arm of Clitoris
Labia majora
Bulb of Clitoris

Frontal view of female reproductive organs

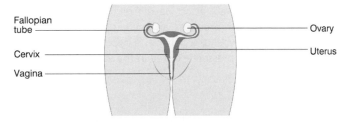

Fallopian tube
Ovary
Cervix
Uterus
Vagina

suggests that this could indeed be a key area in erotic stimulation during intercourse and notes that if the area is not stimulated efficiently, it may be a reason why some women never achieve orgasm from penile thrusting alone during intercourse.

Dr Levin made this first published study of the P-area after monitoring whether the area was drawn into and out of the vaginal opening during intercourse. He used explicit sexual videos, which graphically portrayed sexual intercourse. As the couple made love and the camera zoomed into the genitalia, he freeze-framed the pictures and took measurements of the P-area by tracing it on the TV monitor. He traced the area on partial withdrawal of the penis and on complete insertion into the vagina, and discovered that usually 50% of the area of tissue is drawn into and out of the vagina during intercourse. He suggests that if this area is highly erotically sensitive it could explain why some women can be stimulated to orgasm by penile thrusting alone, but others who have little erotic sensitivity in this area, perhaps because of a biological problem, would find this less stimulating.

'What is needed is a study of the arousal/erotic sensitivity of this area especially in women who claim to have orgasms from coitus alone compared to those who do not. With such a study we may get an answer to the problem why some women have orgasms at coitus and others don't.'

G-spot or G-area

Another highly erotic zone known as the G-spot and perhaps more accurately described as the G-area, is claimed to be a region on the anterior vaginal wall which some women find highly sexually arousing. Before arousal the area is the size of a pea but can enlarge considerably. The area was originally identified in 1950 but did not achieve recognition until the 1980s although it is true to say that not every woman can locate this particularly sensitive area. Indeed, while some women find stimulation of this area highly erotic, others say it is painful and, when stimulated, can make them feel as though they want to urinate, while others feel nothing at all.

It is suggested that the G-spot in the female is equivalent to the prostate in a male: cells in the embryo which develop into the prostate in a man remain small and may become the G-spot in a woman. (It is interesting to note that some men derive pleasure from massage of the prostate gland via the rectum). It has also been suggested that stimulation of the G-spot produces an analgesic effect which is important during childbirth. It is activated when the pelvic and hypogastric nerves are stimulated by the dilation of the cervix and pressure exerted in the vagina by the emerging foetus[3].

The urethra
A FEMALE SEXUAL ORGAN?

During research into the Femidom (the female condom) ultrasound imaging confirmed that during intercourse there is a substantial degree of stretching of the front wall of the vagina and the urethra, as the base of the bladder is pushed backwards by the thrusting penis. (It is interesting that in the original work on the G-spot, the gyneocologist Dr Ernst Graafenberg, after which it was named, found that the urethra was surrounded by erectile tissue, and during sex this enlarged to such a degree that it could be easily felt in the upper wall of the vagina.)

Dr Levin suggests that the stretching of this tissue releases serotonin and other chemicals from cells in the urethral wall – enhancing pleasurable sensations from the urethra during arousal. His conclusion is that during sex the urethra becomes engorged with blood, becoming a sexual organ which can be stimulated and therefore plays a part in sexual arousal which has not yet been widely recognised.

The clitoris

For many – but not all – women the clitoris heightens sexual feelings during intercourse and contributes to increased vaginal lubrication, making sex easier and more pleasurable. The clitoris contains thousands of nerve endings making it highly sensitive and as women age the clitoris increases in size.

A women with a poorly developed clitoris experiences low levels of sexual interest, says Dr Levin. She experiences sexual arousal and achieves orgasm with difficulty. Testosterone treatment can improve clitoral size and sensitivity and trials have shown that treating women with androgens can help. However it is recognised that some women do not get clitoral stimulation during intercourse and some women report that they receive no pleasurable sensation from the clitoris, that it is effectively 'numb' or 'dead'. So, although the clitoris has long been thought of as the principal key to pleasure for sex for women, it may only be a part of the story.

The Australian urologist Helen O'Connell published a paper published in 1998, in which she said that that the internal part of the clitoris is about three times the size it is portrayed in *Gray's Anatomy*, the anatomist's bible. The true size of the clitoris has always been hidden away inside women and this new information should be useful for surgeons performing pelvic surgery on women. O'Connell became aware as a urology trainee that she had to take special care while removing the prostate in men with prostate cancer to ensure that everything was done to preserve their sexual function. She found that no one had ever undertaken a detailed investigation of the clitoris and the nerves that supply it, although Japanese doctors have developed a centre of excellence in this field.

O'Connell's description of the clitoris is that the external tip connects on the inside to a large, pyramid shaped mass of erectile tissue. The suggestion is that the clitoris surrounds the urethra, the P-spot and the vaginal cavity.

The shaft of the clitoris is about as big as the joint of a thumb. This has two arms which flare up backwards into the body. Also extending

> **FACT:**
>
> The clitoris was first accurately described in 1559 and the term first appears in English in 1615, according to Dr Levin.

from the clitoris and filling the space between its arms are two bulbs one on each side of the vaginal cavity.

Most textbooks do not connect these areas together, referring to them as the bulbs of the vestibule. Rather than the clitoris being separate from the urethra, she has found that it is, in fact, connected on three sides, which adds weight to what previous researchers have already found. This, O'Connell believes, helps to squeeze the urethra shut during intercourse. Furthermore, the cavernosal nerves thought to control the muscles of the clitoris travel alongside the wall of the urethra, vagina, bladder and urethra. During sex the clitoris enlarges in both length and diameter due to blood flow and engorgement.

The labia

The labia are folds of skin which contain fatty tissue and a thin layer of smooth muscle similar to the muscle fibres of the male scrotum. They also contain erogenous tissue that can become engorged, especially the *labia minora*. During arousal the labia lift and flattens as they engorge with blood. The direct parallel to the labia is the scrotum of men.

The cervix

Although the cervix has no 'sexual feeling' it may play a part in stimulating other erotically sensitive areas. Dr Levin says: 'When the cervix is jostled by the penis during intercourse some women claim that the rubbing of the uterus (via the cervix against the lining membrane at the peritoneum) gives them pleasurable sexual feelings.' Women who have hysterectomies involving the loss of the cervix do sometimes report a loss or a reduction of sexual feeling.

The vagina

Some women say that pressure on the muscles running around the vagina also gives them a pleasurable feeling. Having sex strengthens the vagina and Dr Levin says there is truth in the old adage 'use it or lose it'. 'Just having intercourse maintains the function of the vagina – it needs exercise, as all muscles do.'

The vagina connects the womb with the external genital organs and is designed to accommodate an erect penis (as well as an emerging baby's head during childbirth). There are three layers of inter- connected tissues:

- a mucous membrane containing large blood vessels, which is influenced by hormonal changes
- smooth muscle richly supplied with blood vessels which swells upon sexual stimulation and which also contains oestrogen receptor cells
- a fibrous layer consisting of collagen and elastin which provides support but can allow expansion of the vagina during intercourse

Blood supply to the vagina is provided by the internal iliac artery, the uterine artery and the pudendal arteries. Contrary to popular belief, the vagina itself is a poor source of erotic arousal because the inner walls are relatively insensitive to the touch. It may be that the amount of pressure applied is the key.

Light pressure has little or no effect. Deep pressure can be sensuously stimulating if the conditions are right and there is no vaginal dryness and no pain – it may in effect stimulate the erectile tissues of the urethra positioned just behind the vaginal walls (and possibly the P- and G-spot areas). Lubrication is vital for painless intercourse and this depends on how good engorgement of the vagina is – which in turn depends on free unrestricted blood flow.

The lubricant or plasma-like material passes through the tiny blood vessels in the vaginal walls and forms sweat-like droplets on the surface during sexual arousal. Chemical messengers innervate blood vessels, triggering the blood flow into the vagina. The engorgement of the vagina raises the pressure inside the capillaries under the surface of the vaginal walls, which allows more of the lubricant to leak through onto the vaginal surface. When sexual stimulation stops, the blood flow lessens and the lubricant stops being produced. The excess fluid is reabsorbed by the outer part of the vagina through active sodium reabsorption and osmosis.

How does this happen?

A neurotransmitter called VIP (vasoactive intestinal peptide which is present in nerves that innervate blood vessels in the vaginal wall) is believed to be the principle trigger for the changes in the vagina (blood flow, lubrication) which occur at arousal. Studies have shown that when VIP is injected intravenously or through an injection into the vaginal wall, vaginal blood increases – and so does lubrication – although it seems to have no effect on feelings of sexual arousal.

The vagus or 'wandering' nerve

Research[3] by scientists at Rutgers University, New Jersey, USA, has found that in women the vagus nerve (that travels through the back and chest) is a 'sensory pathway' from the vagina and cervix directly to the brain.

(The word vagus means wandering, and the nerve supplies a whole host of organs: it plays a part in digestion, yawning and sneezing and to supply the lungs and heart, among other functions.)

The work by Dr Beverly Whipple and Prof. Barry Komisaruk provides a rational explanation for the phenomenon that women who have suffered complete spinal cord injury can nevertheless experience sexual responses including orgasm. The vagus nerve provides an alternative route into the brain, by-passing the spinal cord, and may explain why some women with spinal cord injuries can also experience menstrual cramps, or labour pains if they have children.

Whipple and Komisaruk's research proves that women with severe spinal injuries can still enjoy orgasm. How and why will reveal important information for all women as we learn more about the different nerves that may feed signals from the genitals to the brain.

The pair have also made the first important discoveries about the different brain regions that are activated during orgasm, by taking special brain scans. This will have repercussions for women who may have an abnormal or damaged nerve pathway and report a loss of sexual drive or loss of sexual feeling, as well as deepening our understanding of the basic neuroscience of sexual experiences.

What can go wrong?

BLOOD FLOW

With such a mass of erectile tissue it is easy to understand how important normal blood circulation is to the genitals if the physiological side of sexual arousal is to work. The focus of some clinicians testing anti-impotence drugs for women is to find the causes of restricted blood flow, and the physiological switches for that necessary blood flow. It may be that drugs currently being tested such as apomorphine and phentalomine work by improving the blood flow upon sexual stimulation once other psychological barriers to good sex are overcome.

Prof. Irwin Goldstein and Dr Jennifer Berman, of Boston University, identified two distinct syndromes:

- abnormal vaginal engorgement and enlargement required for intercourse. Symptoms: delayed vaginal engorgement, lack of orgasm, or low orgasmic sensation
- clitoral erectile insufficiency syndrome. Symptoms: diminished clitoral sensation and orgasm

They summarise: 'There is a growing body of evidence that women with sexual dysfunction will commonly have physiologic abnormalities such as female sexual dysfunction, due to impaired blood flow, contributing to their overall sexual health problems.' Decreased blood flow may affect the sexual sensations by affecting the release of nitric oxide and cause atrophy and collapse of nerve fibres and cells lining the vaginal canal and inner labia, according to Dr Berman (see box on page 51). Pelvic arterial disease may cause arteries to fur up, restricting blood flow to the genitals.

NOTE:

Work at the Centre d'Etudes des Dysfonctions Sexuelles in Lyons, France, reported at the Eighth World Meeting on Impotence Research in Amsterdam in August 1998, shows that clitoral blood flow increases during stimulation of the lower part of the vagina by between 4 and 11 times the pre-stimulation level. The results they suggested, are the same as recorded in the cavernous arteries in men when pressure is applied to the penis. This, the researchers conclude, suggests a sexual synergy between partners in which vascular and muscular responses mirror each other and are reciprocally reinforced during intercourse.

Research in America suggests that risk factors for this problem include:
- high blood pressure
- smoking
- obesity
- coronary artery disease
- diabetes
- high cholesterol levels
- bicycle riding – a urologist in New Jersey has found that in a study of 282 female cyclists, more than 40% reported clitoral numbness

HOPE FOR WOMEN WITH SPINAL CORD INJURIES

Sex can still be enjoyed
Researchers at the Kessler Institute for Rehabilitation in West Orange, New Jersey, conducted a survey into the sexual responses of women with spinal cord injuries. Twenty-five affected women took part in the trial and 52% of them were able to achieve orgasm regardless of the pattern or degree of neurological injury. It was noted that women who achieved orgasms had a higher sex drive and greater sexual knowledge. Women involved in another study on the sexual response of women with spinal injuries said they felt a conscious awareness of shutting out sexuality because of their injury – largely because they assumed that sexual pleasure was no longer possible in the absence of genital sensation. They expressed a sense of worthlessness and avoided engaging in sex with partners. However, many found that their sexual interest did return with the support of a communicative, open partner although it may have been a long while after the accident. Research now proves it is possible to resume a sex life with a grave spinal injury which gives hope to affected women.
One extraordinary finding is that the vagus nerve can in some women, be stimulated from other parts of the body – one woman in the trials experienced an orgasm after applying a vibrator to her neck and shoulders. The research has also shown that the body releases oxytocin and prolactin during orgasm – oxytocin increases pleasure during sex and promotes nurturing feelings or 'bonding' between sexual partners.
Dr Whipple and Prof. Komisaruk sum up their attitudes to female sexuality with some good advice for both women and doctors on the threshold of achieving greater understanding and acceptance of sexuality and sexual problems.
'Whatever the final outcome in terms of neural pathways and neurotransmitters involved in sexual response it is important for physicians to be aware of the variety of sexual response that women report and that have been documented in the laboratory.
'It is also important for women to be aware of what is pleasurable to them, to acknowledge this to themselves and then to communicate what they find pleasurable to their partners.
'People need to be encouraged to feel good about the variety of ways they may achieve sexual pleasure without setting up specific goals (e.g. finding the G-spot or experiencing female ejaculation). 'Healthy sexuality begins with acceptance of the self, in addition to an emphasis on the process, rather than only the goals, of sexual interaction.'
From *Medical Aspects of Human Sexuality*, June 1998

Drugs which may influence sexual arousal are:
- antihistamines
- antihypertensives
- antidepressants
- antipsychotics
- antioestrogens
- central nervous system stimulants
- narcotics
- alcohol

Some drugs prescribed for depression and high blood pressure can affect mood and also the blood supply or response of the tissues. It's thought that nearly half the patients who take tricyclic antidepressants like clomipramine can experience FSD.

A study on the effects of propranol, the commonly prescribed drug for hypertension and angina, in 1990 by Alan Riley, found that it significantly affected sexual arousal in nine healthy young women. Ace inhibitors and calcium channel blockers may have an impact on libido.

Drugs for depression can also affect women's sexual function notably their ability to attain orgasm, or a delay in reaching orgasm,– and these include Prozac (fluoxetine), sertraline, and paroxetine from a group of drugs called selective serotonin reuptake inhibitors or SSRIs. Dramatic effects on desire and arousal, and genital numbness have been reported by some women taking SSRIs. One report in the US suggests that 33% of women who use SSRIs will experience loss of libido and difficulty in achieving orgasm.

Sedatives may also have an impact – even commonly available products such as

---

NOTE:

In men nitric oxide is the key to penile erections – the fuel for sex. At arousal the endothelial cells that line the penis start manufacturing more and more which triggers a muscle-relaxing chemical (cGMP) but an enzyme called PDE5 impedes this process. Viagra works by blocking the PDE5 enzyme allowing blood to flow into the corpus cavernosum of the penis, and an erection to occur. Preliminary studies suggest that nitric oxide is also important in the engorgement of clitoral tissues in women. Prof. Goldstein believes a similar process is at work in women: research in animals has shown that if there is arterial insufficiency to the clitoris it can stop the engorgement of erectile tissues thus reducing sexual sensation. It is likely that blood needs to travel unimpeded to the clitoris and all the erectile tissues surrounding the urethra, Prof. Goldstein and Dr Berman, a urologist and director of Boston University's Women's Sexual Health Clinic, presented their theory that some women can experience sexual dysfunction due to impaired blood flow to an international conference at Cape Cod, USA on May 30, 1998 and published a scientific paper in the International Journal of Impotence Research 10, supplement 2.

Valium. Prescribed to relieve anxiety, they can also cause loss of sexual desire and arousal problems.

Contraceptives and other drugs

Progesterone dominant pills may cause the most complaints of loss of sexual interest. Combined oral contraception (COC) is known to decrease serum testosterone levels by decreasing ovarian production of testosterone and increasing production of sex hormone-binding globulin (SHBG) from the liver. Until recently it was thought that levels return to normal once a woman stops taking COC. However, in a study of 102 women with sexual dysfunction, researchers from Boston University School Medicine found that levels of SHBG can remain elevated for up to a year after stopping COC.

The Kinsey Institute in America has also studied the effects of oral contraceptives on sexual interest, response and mood. Researchers found that after taking oral contraceptives for three months, levels of testosterone, free testosterone (FT) and the hormone DHEA fell in all 61 women who took part, although the extent of the reduction was variable. Some women reported a decrease in frequency of sexual thoughts but others experienced no loss of sexual interest in spite of substantial reduction in FT and there was overall no evidence that reduction in FT affected enjoyment of sexual activity with a partner.

The findings were consistent with the idea that some women may be more sensitive to changes in testosterone than others. Researchers concluded that what distinguishes women who experience negative sexual side effects as a result of reduced testosterone levels from those who do not remains unexplained and a question of crucial importance for future research.

In 1986, a study[4] by Prof. Alan Riley found that some women's sexual feelings, and the time it takes to reach orgasm, may be affected by diazepam. One of the women involved in the trial was unable to reach orgasm at all. It is thought that the drug might impair the necessary psychological input required for the feelings of sexual desire.

Tamoxifen, the drug often prescribed to women after breast cancer, may cause vaginal bleeding and discharge which may lead to a lack of interest in sex.

Diseases and disorders which may have an effect upon female sexual arousal

Diabetes is a known cause of impotence in men – and doctors are now looking at the consequences in women. Diabetes affects nerves and blood vessels throughout the body and can affect the circulation of the blood and damage pathways which, as we have already seen, play a vital role in sending signals of pleasure from the genitals to the brain.

A possible complication of diabetes is hardening and narrowing of the arteries, which could affect blood supply to the genital area. As clitoral insufficiency may be caused by a restricted blood flow it is possible that a diabetic woman may lose some genital sensation.

Thyroid problems are another cause of loss of sexual desire; either an underactive thyroid (the condition is called hypothyroidism) or an overactive thyroid (hyperthyroidism) can influence sexual feelings (*see case history on page 55*). The thyroid is a vital gland, influencing body weight, energy levels, skin condition, mental state, reproductive organs and also sexual functioning.

There are worries that many women with hypothyroidism go undiagnosed because its symptoms of depression, mood swings and muscle weakness are often confused with other problems such as menopause or stress. The condition can, however, be diagnosed with a blood test. Women over 40 are at greatest risk from thyroid disorders.

Women who have thyroid disease may have a testosterone deficiency. An overactive thyroid increases the amount of sex hormone binding globulin which controls the amount of testosterone available in the body and can lead to a deficiency. Without this vital sex drive fuel you can experience a loss of libido and desire.

Links between high blood pressure and sexual problems in women were first made in 1997. A study by Dr Laurie Gordon presented to the American Heart Association's 70th scientific sessions in Florida in November made the connection. The main problems reported were difficulty in achieving orgasm and inadequate vaginal lubrication.

Oestrogen protects women from heart disease until the menopause – when levels fall women become as susceptible as men. In men, the same deposits which cause arteries of the heart to fur up also occur in the arteries of the pelvis which supplies the penis. A small number of women suffering from heart disease may develop the same condition leading to a restricted blood supply in the pelvis.

If you have had a heart attack you may be fearful about resuming sex – but the British Heart Foundation say it should be fine two to three weeks after a heart attack. If you get pain during sex talk to your doctor.

Surgery and sex

Having pelvic surgery or radiation therapy in the pelvic area can sometimes result in vaginal discomfort and even sexual dysfunction. Sexual problems are common among women who have had cervical or endometrial surgery.

Hysterectomy will compromise production of oestrogen, progesterone and androgen, which all play a part in sex drive and arousal. There is still little guidance for surgeons on the nerves which control sexual response but some are receiving specialised training in nerve-sparing techniques in Japan.

Many women who have had hysterectomies and removal of the cervix frequently report a reduction in sexual feelings and response after radical surgery. This often does not show until a year or so after surgery. During the first year women may benefit from the relief of symptoms – such as heavy periods due to fibroids, or freedom from severe and painful periods – and go through a honeymoon period. It is not until later that the

CASE HISTORY

Frances Quirk staged some of the first large-scale research into FSD for Pfizer. And two years into the project she discovered her own sexual drive had 'evaporated'.
Frances' work involves plenty of international travel. On a 10-day trip to Australia she took melatonin – a supplement available in the US but not the UK – to combat jet lag.
But on her return she suffered what she described as an 'acute episode of strange symptoms'.
'I was forgetting things, I was using the wrong word in a sentence, my skin got dry and my hair fell out and my sex drive totally disappeared.
'It was just fortunate that I had a health check booked at work and it turned out that my thyroid function was abnormally low.'
All Frances' symptoms were linked to a condition called hypothyroidism.
The most worrying was losing her desire for sex which she described as 'something just switching off'.
'I had a particular good sex drive – my husband and I had been together for four or five years before this and unless we were away or had guests we would have sex each day,' she said. 'I was a normal, healthy sexual person.'
Losing that drive came as a total shock, she said.
'It was really something that I defined myself by. It meant 'this is me', this is what I am, this is part of me. It was like having a particular personality.
'It was like someone trying to communicate with you in a fog – or someone trying to say something to you that had no meaning at all.'
Frances found it upsetting because she had

enjoyed a good relationship with husband Iain – and the couple had instigated sex, equally.
'My husband thought I had had an affair in Australia because the change in me had been so dramatic – my sex drive had evaporated completely. Any feeling I would have had in response to my husband's advances was just gone.'
Frances continued her sexual relationship with her husband but she said it was not the same. 'That was really rather shocking.'
But she knew deep down she had not fallen out of love with her husband and that her loving feelings were the same. Fortunately the couple were able to talk it through and she was able to explain that there was a physiological explanation.
But she knows it was hard for her husband to understand and she believes this is because men so rarely lose that desire.
Fortunately Frances and her doctor were able to link her loss of sex drive with her thyroid condition, which was diagnosed fairly quickly after her return from Australia and this helped Iain to understand her problem better.
She knows she is fortunate and that some women she has interviewed continued to suffer this sort of loss for years.
Frances has been treated with thyroxine – but she knows that her low thyroid functioning can still affect her. But it took two and half years for things to resolve.
'My sexual desire is the chief marker for me now – there is a very direct relationship for me between low thyroid levels and my loss of desire.'
Even now Frances knows her sexual drive is not the same as it once was.
'I suppose it's functioning at about 70% of what I expect but it is something that I now have to live with.'

long-term effects may be felt.

Dr Cees Maas, a research fellow in gynaecological oncology at Leiden University, Holland, has studied nerve-sparing surgical techniques for cervical cancer operations at the National Cancer Centre, the National Cancer Hospital, and the Juntendo University Hospital, in Japan.

Maas worked on the first study[5] to look at the vaginal blood flow response during sexual stimulation after hysterectomy and found that women who had undergone radical hysterectomies had significantly lower responses. This suggests that surgery without due attention to nerves supplying blood vessels to the vaginal wall can lead to sexual problems in terms of arousal and lubrication. He told a major international conference in Canada in 2002: 'Women with a history of surgery for cervical cancer report decreased lubrication and genital swelling during sexual arousal which compromises sexual activity and results in considerable distress.'

Some women report that although they experience orgasms, these are not as strong as they were before the operation. More recently, research published in the British Journal of Urology showed that after radical surgery for superficial bladder cancer or invasive carcinoma, 45 per cent of women reported diminished ability or inability to achieve orgasm, 41 per cent reported decreased lubrication, 37 per cent decreased sexual desire and 22 per cent painful sex. Only 48 per cent of the 27 patients were able to have successful vaginal intercourse, with 52 per cent reporting decreased satisfaction in overall sexual life.

Dr Beverly Whipple advises raising the issue with your surgeon before an operation. 'Nerve-sparing surgery is now routine for men undergoing pelvic operations, such as pelvic nerve sparing prostatectomy,' she says. 'However, similar surgical procedures do not always exist for women, who are much more likely to undergo pelvic operations such as hysterectomies, which can damage the nerves responsible for the uterine contractions that are an integral aspect of the orgasmic experience.

'Removal of the nerves also affects a woman's response to G spot stimulation. A woman who needs to have a hysterectomy should ask for pelvic nerve sparing and ask to keep her uterine cervix if possible. This helps retain sexual pleasure.'

Influential sex hormones

ANDROGENS (TESTOSTERONE)

Testosterone is produced by women in small amounts and is thought to be a key hormone in sex drive. This makes sense as the tissue of woman's genitals are androgen-dependent. The clitoris, labia probably the P-spot and even pubic hair and nipples are all androgen-dependent.

As men mature they lose androgen receptors in the penis, but as women age they don't lose receptors in the clitoris. However, levels of testosterone gradually drop: women in their 40s produce roughly half the amount of women in their 20s. Some

DIAGNOSTIC EQUIPMENT

A breakthrough in research into women's sexual problems has come through an ability to monitor changes in vaginal blood flow, and the development of clinical questionnaires in which women 'self report' their problems.

These machines work in a similar way to biofeedback devices. They are used to monitor changes in the engorgement of the vagina, labia or clitoris with blood when women are shown erotic images or are asked to indulge in sexual fantasy, and they feed back information about that woman's physiological state of sexual arousal.

The problem is that these devices may not be as accurate in a laboratory as they are in a real sexual situation at home, although they will undoubtedly register changes and that may be enough to provide a measure of sexual arousal.

A simple subjective rating scale (when a woman is asked to rate her level of arousal from 1-10) has flaws: some women find this interferes with arousal and the levels may vary from one woman to another.

Sometimes women say they are unable to become aroused – but in fact do. Biofeedback can help teach a woman recognise the signs of arousal (see *chapter eleven – adjustments to your sex life*).

women have been helped to regain sensitivity in the genitals by using androgen implants; but it is still considered controversial by some doctors because of possible side-effects (*See chapter seven – treatments and chapter eight – testosterone*).

Prolactin and oxytocin

Both these hormones are produced by the pituitary in response to stimulation of the nipples and the genitals. There is much scientific interest in the role of prolactin which has a function in the production of human milk – it is thought that too much of it depresses the sex drive (and it is understood that levels rise at times of stress). This may go some way to explaining why some women are not interested in sex after childbirth and during breast feeding.

Oestrogen

Oestrogen is important for maintaining the layer of cells in the lining of the vagina. From the menopause, levels of oestrogen fall: and older women can suffer from a condition known as 'vaginal atrophy' where the lining of the vagina diminishes. With fewer blood vessels supplying the vagina it becomes more difficult to lubricate. However, older women still have the ability to lubricate but may need more stimulation.

An alternative to HRT may be found in a diet rich in phytoestrogens which have an uncanny ability to mimic natural oestrogen in the body but are only fractionally as potent as the human kind. It is thought that phytoestrogens are able to compete for receptor sites and block the uptake of excess oestrogen and may be able to protect against hormonally induced cancers (see *chapter five – sex and the menopause*).

Progesterone

This is also a sex hormone which balances the effects of oestrogen. Diet, stress and the menopause can all affect progesterone production which, in turn, can lead to tiredness and decreased libido. Natural progesterone creams which are rubbed into the fatty areas of the body, mimic the effects of progesterone in the body and claims are made that this can help to improve a flagging sex drive .

Equipment used

- Doppler ultra-sonography measures blood speed and movement in the clitoral cavernosal artery and has been used to record changes associated with stimulating the vagina. The study found that blood velocity increased 11 times that of the pre-stimulation pattern.
- Vaginal photo-plethysmography involves shining an infra-red light into the vaginal tissue and recording the amount reflected back. More infrared light is reflected back to a photosensitive sensor as vaginal engorgement increases. The greater the blood content of the vaginal walls, the more the amount of reflected light.
- Heat wash out or 'vaginal thermal clearance' is a more accurate measurement, which involves a heated electrode held in position within a gold, silver or platinum disc. As blood flow increases due to sexual arousal, more heat is transferred away from the heated device and more electrical power is needed to maintain the electrode at a fixed temperature. Higher amounts of energy indicate higher levels of blood flow and, it is inferred, higher levels of sexual arousal.

Food for thought:

Roy Levin[6] makes the point that when all goes well, human lovers have 'an all-consuming passion for one another'. The heat of desire eventually cools, and, for some, sexual desire for a partner fades and becomes extinct. Levin questions whether sexual desire is dependent on a barrier or difference between people that needs to be overcome and that when closeness is too great the two partners 'fuse into one and there are no differences to overcome'.

Yet while easy access kills passion and weakens desire, no access at all will also eventually kill passion. Such subtleties and complexities of human sexual desire make it one of the hardest dysfunctions to treat. 'It is not too difficult to see why there is so much current interest in . . . pharmacological treatments to enhance female sexual arousal. Humans always hope for a magic pill to cure their ills!'

Further information and help:

Diabetes UK, Macleod House, 10 Parkway, London, NW1 7AA.
Tel: 020 7424 1000 www.diabetes.org.uk
The association also runs a Careline open Monday to Friday from 9am to 5pm: 0845 1202960

or e-mail careline@diabetes.org.uk

British Heart Foundation, *14 Fitzhardinge Street, London, W1H 4DH.*
Tel: 0207 9350185   *www.bhf.org.uk*

Outsiders *A group campaigning for the acceptance of disabled people as sexual partners.*
Tel 0207 354 8291   *www.outsiders.org.uk*
The group runs a Sex and Disability Helpline open 11am to 7pm Monday to Friday: 0707 4993527

References

[1]Levin, R. The physiology of sexual arousal in the human female: a recreational and procreational synthesis. *Archives of Sexual Behavior* 2002. **31** (5): 405-411.
[2]Sexual Appetite, Desire and Motivation: Energetics of the Sexual System, publ. Royal Netherlands Academy of Arts and Sciences, 2001
[3]Whipple, B., Komisaruk, B. Beyond the G-Spot: recent research on female sexuality. *Medical Aspects of Human Sexuality* 1998. **1** (3): 19-23.
Tepper, M., Whipple, B., Richard, E., Komisaruk, B. R. Women with complete spinal cord injury: a phenomenological study of sexual experiences. *Journal of Sex and Marital Therapy* 2001. **27**: 615-623.
Whipple, B., Komisaruk, B. R. Sexuality and women with complete spinal cord injury. *Spinal Cord* 1997. **35**: 136-138
[4]Riley, A. *Journal of Sexual and Marital Therapy* 1986, Vol. 1 No. 1.
[5]Disturbance of Vaginal Blood Flow after uterine surgery, psychophysiological study, CP Maas, ISSWSH annual meeting, Vancouver October 10-13, 2002.
[6]Levin, R. Sexual Desire and the Deconstruction and Reconstruction of the Human Female Sexual Response Model of Masters and Johnson. **In**: Everard, W., Laan, E., Both, S. (eds) A Sexual appetite, desire and motivation: energetics of the sexual system, pp. 63-93. The Royal Academy of Arts and Sciences, Amsterdam, 2001.

4

sex and the mind

'I cannot separate my sexual being from my emotional being – having a problem with sexual arousal has ruined my marriage. It definitely affects me a great deal because I have very little sexual desire and it is related to pain, making me generally unhappy. It is very hard to have a good relationship with a man when there is no sexual relationship there.'
Eve, aged 27

Counselling will help if you have a deep-seated psychological or behavioural reason for your sexual difficulties. Counselling won't help if your problem is a physical one which would need addressing first. After treatment you may still require some help from a sex therapist if the biological problem was long-standing and has led to an aversion to sex.

The way psychosexual counselling is offered in the UK is changing.
Jane Roy, head of Relate's psycho-sexual therapy service, says counsellors are more prepared to refer a woman to a health professional or doctor than in the past. This is because therapists are much more aware of the possibility that sex problems may be linked to medical ones. She says some 50% of cases now fall into this category. So, just as doctors refer their patients to Relate, now around 17% of cases are referred by therapists to doctors. 'We ensure more than we used to that clients are checked out medically,' she says.

In the past – and it may still happen with some independent counsellors – women have become needlessly anxious and concerned by being questioned about their childhood sexual experiences when, in fact, they have been suffering a long-term organic problem (such as a hormonal imbalance) which was causing their sexual difficulty. This can affect the partner's feelings: if psychotherapy fails to work he may feel utterly rejected, and it may also result in you feeling desperate because your problem cannot be solved.

A survey by Relate has found that during 2001 more people have been accessing sex therapy than ever before – and it is mainly women who make the first contact. The survey of nearly 200 sex therapists found that 508 couples sought help – but also 50 lone women. The most common age of women seeking help at Relate is between 30 and 39, closely followed by the 18-to-29 age group.

Jane Roy, who organised the survey, says Relate's sex therapy clients are no longer exclusively heterosexual couples – 14% of clients are now coming alone or with a same sex partner. The most common disorders involved desire problems – but more than 30% of couples had more than one sexual dysfunction. The desire problems can arise for many different reasons. In one case a woman's husband suffered a heart attack – and she lost her desire for sex because she became fearful for her husband's health. 'It was a way of protecting him,' explains Ms Roy.

But there are other subtle pressures that can put women off sex. She says: 'One of the issues that causes the most problems with couples in a committed relationship is the feeling they have 'got' to have intercourse. It can help to say 'no'. You don't have to fall into the trap of having intercourse each time.' Also, she says there are some couples who simply don't have a high sex drive – but that is 'normal' for them and they just need reassuring.

Using techniques such as sensate focus, which sets aside allotted time for non-genital contact at first, can relieve some of those pressures. She concludes: 'The overall evidence from this study is that Relate therapists are still dealing with a full range of sexual dysfunctions. They see clients from teenagers to pensioners. In a third of cases they have creatively to combine treatment strategies for more than one dysfunction. Nearly half of their cases involve medical issues of some kind and so they are having to adapt treatment programmes to accommodate health issues.'

Health problems recorded in the survey ranged from diabetes to endometriosis, and vaginismus after childbirth. Depression and drug treatment for it were frequent medical issues and the report stated: 'It is well known that depression and some of the treatments for depression can lead to a sexual problem.'

In other cases, the link seemed more associated with the psychological consequences of an illness rather than its direct physical consequences – such as loss of desire associated with irritable bowel or Crohn's disease. There was even one case where both partners were experiencing loss of desire and the therapist recorded under 'medical issues': 'health problems of their child.' Ms Roy concludes: 'More research is needed into the relationship between illness and sexual dysfunction in a couple's relationship.'

Sex therapists are trained counsellors and psychotherapists. Some can undertake medical examinations of women but most cannot. However, if they feel it is the right course of action, they will work in conjunction with a GP or specialist. Dr Kevan Wylie, director of the Porterbrook Clinic in Sheffield and an NHS doctor treating patients with sexual problems for 25 years, says one of the challenges of the future will be separating out women who have sex drive problems (more biologically based) and sexual desire problems (more emotional or psychological) and then treating them accordingly.

At present there are a number of NHS centres able to offer this form of combined approach. One of them is the Jane Wadsworth Clinic at St Mary's Hospital in London. A study involving 47 women who attended the sexual dysfunction clinic over a period of three months divided patients into different groups depending on whether they saw a doctor, a psychologist, a doctor and a psychologist, or a sex therapist. All therapists attempted to assess the success rate of their treatment but this was only possible in the case of 32 of the patients. Although the figures are low they are interesting:

The rates of success were:
- seeing a physician: 100% (although it was only 3/3)
- seeing a psychologist: 66.6%
- seeing a physician and psychologist together (conjoint clinic): 83.3%
- seeing a sexual therapist: 75%

How sex therapy works
Relate has around 200 sex therapists at different regional centres, and is the country's major provider of sex therapy. A survey carried out in 1996 revealed that around 40% of couples now 'self refer' to Relate and as many as 75% have a successful outcome. Sex therapists tend to focus on couples' therapy and sensate focus, a programme of exercises done at home which can uncover deep relationship problems or abnormal feelings about sex.

Some therapists will see women, or men alone and work out individual sensate focus programmes for them. Couples' therapy is fine for people who are in long-term relationships and need help but not effective for women whose problems have a biological basis. Sex therapy, however, certainly has a place in the treatment of women's sexual problems: an inability to want to participate in sexual intercourse frequently has a psychological cause, which can be improved with therapy. But it can only improve your sex life if there are anxieties or worries or misplaced thoughts that need help or correcting. It will also only work if there is still an intact sex drive and a strong wish for an improved sex life.

It is surprising how many couples simply don't know anything about sexual process and even their genitalia. Therapists now use pictures and diagrams to spell it all out. 'There is a lot of ignorance – a lot of women and men still don't really know where the clitoris is or what its function is. This is sex education for adults – in its broadest sense,' says Ms Roy.

According to psychologists we are all born with an in-built sensitivity to sexual stimuli – this is our arousability factor. This arousability is influenced by our memories and our experiences, our attraction to our partner and also physiological conditions such as healthy nerves and the right flow of chemicals to transmit sensation to the brain.

Sex drive is said to be the strongest natural drive after hunger and sleep. This arousability factor inevitably changes as we age and have more experience of life. It is also a mechanism which can be affected by over-familiarisation – in other words having sex with the same person, perhaps in the same position in the same situation year after year, can be a major passion killer.

In addition, relationships change over the years and this can influence how we 'see' our lovers. Partners might become more child-like because of age or ill-health and the relationship might transfer from a sexual one to a nurturing one.

Taking the first step

The hurdle you may face is overcoming embarrassment. Although the taboos for seeking treatment for sexual problems are at last being broken down, it still may not be easy for you to talk about yourself until more clinics become 'women friendly' and are set up especially to help women and their specific and increasing needs. But bear in mind that professional sex therapists are trained to understand this feeling of embarrassment and will help you. They should make the interview and therapy sessions as comfortable as possible. Be prepared to see two therapists working as a team. The idea is to widen the perspective and some clinics like the idea of one therapist chaperoning another. If you don't want two therapists in on the session, ask whether it is OK to see just one, as there are plenty who prefer to operate on their own.

The psychological problems

There may be a temporary aversion to sex because of depression, anxiety, anger, miscarriage, overbearing family responsibilities, money worries or bereavement. Or the problem may be more deep rooted and be associated with rape, childhood abuse, parental or religious influences. Growing up in a family with strong sexual taboos can lead to sexual dysfunction, and problems with orgasm. This can lead to feelings of distress because you feel unable to please your partner, resulting in a vicious circle of anxiety, decreased lubrication and pain on intercourse and leading eventually to sexual avoidance and relationship breakdown. Depression – or drugs given to treat it – may also play a part, along with a loss of self- confidence and self-esteem.

A study by the Kinsey Institute has found that women with depressive mood symptoms have significantly lower sexual desire than women with normal mood. A UK study has also found that six per cent of women questioned about their sexual difficulties were depressed. Traditionally women who have lost their confidence or esteem or suffer from depression may be unable to reach orgasm – something switches off before climax, perhaps associated with a fear of letting go and losing control (see *chapter ten – the happiness factor*).

These factors can negatively influence the mind which holds the power of an 'override switch' to sex. Negative thoughts, worries and distractions can all bring sexual feelings to a sudden halt. Therapy can help put fears into perspective or enable women to change their response by learning to exchange the negative idea that sex is bad in some way for more positive thoughts and feelings.

Key psychological problems affecting sexual arousal:
- anxiety
- mood
- anger

The sexual circuitry
What goes on in the mind and in the emotions will strongly influence the 'sexual reflex', say sex therapists. Sexual arousal can be compared to an electrical circuit – which can be subject to breakdowns at many different junctions along the route to sexual fulfillment.

The break points are:
- pain – which can cancel out sexual response
- emotional interference with the sexual response – anxiety, sadness, grief, bereavement, anger
- distraction – fear of pregnancy, negative memories, uncertainty as to how to behave. In psycho-speak some women can suffer from 'spectatoring': you are too busy worrying, and using your mind's eye to 'see' or 'watch' what you are doing to allow yourself to be carried along with your sexual feelings to the exclusion of all else

The impact of loss of sexual feelings
Women whose lives have been blighted by problems with sexual arousal feel guilty, less good about themselves, and experience a sense of their loss at a part of their lives they once enjoyed to the full. The problem not only affects them individually, in the way they feel about themselves, but also touches others around them, notably husbands and families. Losing touch with sexuality and sexual feelings can result

> **NOTE:**
>
> There is a subtle difference between psychotherapy and sex therapy: sex therapists work on the physical responses as well as the mental responses. Therefore sex therapy is not just 'all talk' – exercises and tasks are set to find out more about the physical blocks and problems, and they can also be used to take the pressure off one or both partners while these problems are explored. A psychotherapist will encourage you to talk more about your problems, and your past which may throw some light on the way you feel.

in stress and tension underscoring much of their lives. 'Sometimes I become angry,' says one woman.'We have rows about it because my partner thinks that I am cold,' says another.

The women quoted below are from Australia, America, the UK, Denmark, France and Italy who talked to researchers about their sexual arousal problems for between 40 and 90 minutes. These sexual difficulties were by and large going untreated – even if they had found a clinician they may not have found a workable treatment – and was affecting their overall quality of life. The most common expression was of a loss, something fundamental missing from their lives, or that an important part of themselves as women had somehow disappeared leaving a hole in their lives.

The negative feelings, they said, directly affected relationships around them, inevitably mostly with their husband although some women spoke of their lack of sexual fulfillment as touching other areas of their lives. Several worried that their partners would leave them, others kept quiet about the pain of sex – the bleeding, discomfort and burning sensations caused by a lack of lubrication or inability to become sexually aroused.

'Sex is an important part of our relationship for him – but it was a while before I realised that he felt that way. He suggested that I see someone but I said it was normal, I was just tired and there would be nothing a doctor could do. As a result he feels slightly rejected and sometimes becomes angry,'
– Ellen, in her 30s, suffering from arousal disorder and lack of interest.

Living with a husband who does not understand his partner's sexual problems adds tension to a marriage.
'It concerns me because it concerns him – it has really become an issue between us,'
– Geraldine, in her 30s.

'My husband is more aggressive, critical, irritated and unsatisfied with a lot of things especially not getting 'sexually released',' said one woman. Another said her problems had impacted upon her husband's self-respect which resulted in them not being so close as before and with him 'losing his mood' with her problem affecting his sexual desire for her. The loss of sexual desire or ability to become aroused places a huge strain on women, the interviews revealed.

'I couldn't think of having a relationship without a satisfactory sex life – I could not say to a man: 'you have to be celibate for the rest of your life',' said another.

'To be physical together with a man is very important but I think having an orgasm is not so important. But I couldn't stand it if there was no chance of me getting better,' said Jayne, in her early 30s.

'Sex is very important – but I don't have the desire for it any more,' complained Kate, in her 40s. *'It used to be good but now it seems like he is not interested anymore either.'*
'I have put on weight which has affected my self-esteem. I don't feel so good about myself.'

'I've become passive without feeling – I feel mechanical when having sex, it is not an adventure anymore. I am irritated and frustrated all day and my self-worth and self-acceptance are not good. It is taking up a lot of energy thinking about it and I am not able to feel relaxed in any situation because of it.'

'The physical effect is not there – it makes me worried and upset. I have turned to eating more and I have low self-esteem.'

'It worries me that I can't stand the thought of it, it's unnatural.'

'It's beginning to become an issue between us.'

'You try to avoid it (sex) which isn't helping us. Sometimes I try to grin and bear it which is really hard.'

'When he gets uptight I worry that it could be a reason for him leaving – I was hoping that past 50 he would have forgotten about it.'

These heart-rending expression of unhappiness have not been fully recognised publicly before. Many women reading these extracts will perhaps recognise their own feelings but we hope that this book will show them that there may be a way forward in the very near future. This silent suffering may soon be over, and there will be clinicians, doctors, therapists and possibly treatments available to them soon.

Sex therapy explained

Many therapists will include some explanation of the physiology of sex, the body's 'sexual circuitry' involving the mind and the body's responses, and the well-established stages of sexual arousal through to climax and 'afterglow'.

The message from sex therapists is that sex does not just involve the genitals but also the mind, and that the sexual experience may be influenced by a whole host of other things such as early ideas about sex, past sexual traumas, parental influences, and current life stresses. They will also be influenced by what a woman thinks about herself: whether she has recently undergone the menopause (a loss of her 'femininity'), breast surgery, or even gynaecological procedures. They can all influence body or self-image and consequently have a damaging effect upon sexual response (see *chapter five – sex and the menopause*).

Therapists will try to get to the root of the problem by allowing couples or individuals time to talk about their difficulty, by giving them 'permission' to try new sexual techniques or, in the case of an older couple, providing the reassurance that, yes, sex is normal and desirable later in life.

Relate sex therapists, for example, begin all therapy sessions by an intensive assessment which involves an initial interview, history taking and round-table chat. The aim, says Relate, is to 'ensure that those cases which proceed to treatment have a reasonable chance of completion'.

At this stage therapists may suggest other courses of action (such as a physical examination) or the couple may decide the process is not for them. Margaret Ramage, a sex therapist working privately in central London and also at NHS clinics in Wandsworth and Lambeth, says she always tries to gather as much information as possible, including both family and medical histories. 'Until you ask specifically it does not occur to some women that their hypertension, diabetes or use of alcohol might have an influence on their sexual response.'

Therapy

Most therapists believe relationship and sexual problems are linked. Sometimes a sex problem can be based on a misunderstanding or ignorance and can be resolved quickly – but more complex cases involve guilt or anxiety. Sex guilt is a recognised 'condition' and may have its origins in childhood. Affected women may have problems with orgasm and climax.

The objective of the therapist will be to:
- allow 'space' for talking
- set realistic goals for the individual or couple
- encourage more communication and talking about sexual feelings
- provide reassurance
- give permission to try different techniques
- make specific suggestions – introduce the idea of masturbation or fantasy and give 'permission' to participate in these actions
- help couples communicate more easily between each other

Standard sex therapy involves a sensate focus programme designed to identify obstacles fears or feelings through 'homework' tasks. It was originally devised by Masters and Johnson, the pioneers of sex therapy in the 1960s. If the programme is delivered well it can work very successfully. The programme helps couples find out about their bodies – and what they enjoy or dislike – sexually. Sarah Litvinoff says in the *Relate Guide to Sex*[1], that sensate focus is probably the most intimate thing you can do with a partner – even more so than heat of the moment sex. Not everyone gets on with sensate focus. Some may feel it is too dictatorial, although therapists say couples can benefit if the pressure to perform is taken off. At the start of sensate focus all genital contact is 'banned'.

Stage one: non-sexual touching. The idea is to help you feel more comfortable with your body and its sensual feelings but take the pressure off performing. You are able to touch any part of your partner's body apart from the genitals or in the case of the man, the woman's breasts.

The point of the exercise is to learn to enjoy being touched – or address feelings of dislike. This sort of touching can generate feelings of anger, resentment or bitterness: once they are out in the open, confronted and then talked about they can disappear. 'Repressing these feelings gives them power,' says Margaret Ramage. Part of her job, she says, is to give a woman permission to have these feelings when she is touched in a sexual way.

Three sessions a week are recommended although in most people's busy lives this is unrealistic as each session should take an hour or two to work. You are able to touch each other anywhere except the genitals and experiment by touching parts of the body you have not touched before.

This stage can include kissing. You will be advised to tell your partner if you don't like something, or use a signal such as touching the hand, and to take it in turns to initiate the sessions.

Stage two: involves more communication, actively telling your partner what you do and don't like. The ban on intercourse remains but by this time you should be getting to understand more about your own erogenous zones and recognising your feelings of pleasure or desire.

Stage three: genital touching with hands or mouth is now permitted, as well as the use of body lotions or gels to help enhance feelings of sensuality.

Stage four: involves gradually increasing sexual arousal even as far as orgasm but before penetration.

Stage five: involves intercourse or, in therapy-speak, 'vaginal containment'. This is done very gently without any thrusting, and very

NOTE:

It can be really disturbing to discover that you don't fancy your partner any longer. Work with a therapist might also include teaching you how to have sexual thoughts and fantasies and also individual sensate focus exercises which will help you to experiment with your body on your own.

slowly, which is important for a woman if she has complained of vaginal pain. This then continues with very gentle movements. 'This stage can be highly pleasurable,' says Margaret Ramage. She says she has considerable success with sensate focus although she often finds that couples come to her saying 'we gave up and had intercourse anyway'. This result, she says, is a good outcome.

Others may experience slow progress for several months between the stages of genital and non-genital touching. Jane Roy of Relate said: 'I personally think it's a mistake to keep couples at non-genital touching for too long as this can increase phobic reactions rather than reduce them.

'When there has been abuse or other reasons to be phobic about genital touch then it might take some weeks to get the couple comfortable with genital touching. But usually if the couple need time, I would go slowly between sensual touch (including genitals) and intercourse so they spend some time exploring and being comfortable with each others increasing arousal.' Many people need extra help with fantasy or masturbation techniques. A whole programme can take several months to complete.

It may be useful to remember:

- sex is a natural response if you let it happen
- try to relax as much as possible
- communicate with your partner if it feels good
- protect yourself from things you don't like by moving the hand away or giving a signal

The sexual response – how psychologists study sexual problems

Psychologists studying female sexual arousal in America and the Netherlands have developed a system that incorporates psychology with physiology. It is called the 'psychophysiological' model and, they say, it can reveal how emotional or past problems can affect the sexual response.

With this form of psychological intervention, women are asked how they perceive their sexual response. This is matched up with what happens to her physiologically using biofeedback equipment. The results can throw light on why a woman might be complaining of a loss of sexual desire.

In a typical session a woman complaining of loss of desire or arousal problems might be asked to indicate her 'awareness' of sexual arousal by her feelings of:

- vaginal pulsing or throbbing
- genital tingling
- vaginal wetness
- increased heart rate
- warmth sensations

In response to an erotic stimulus (watching an erotic video, for example) she might be

asked about her feelings of:
- disgust
- anger
- guilt
- anxiety
- enjoyment
- pleasure

A woman who complained of loss of sexual desire might actually have a normal physiological response but somehow their sexual feelings have been transferred to guilt, anxiety or disgust, possibly through a past experience. Affected women may benefit from cognitive behaviour therapy, which would aim to refocus their sexual feelings in a positive way.

An important finding is that many women do not necessarily take into account what is happening to their genitals – they relate sexual arousal to what is happening externally to stimulate them. This is quite different to what happens with men who seem to need the feeling of an erection. The blood flowing into the penis is crucial for their sexual arousal. It is not until later in the sexual arousal cycle that the physiological arousal of lubrication and genital warmth becomes important for a woman.

Note of caution: always ensure that you use a reputable sex therapist. At present there is no law to stop anyone setting themselves up as a 'sex therapist'. Check credentials and look for a therapist who has been accredited by Relate or the British Association of Sexual and Relationship Therapy. If you are interested in surrogate therapy ensure your therapist does not offer him or herself as the surrogate. This is considered unethical.

Further information
Relate's head office is at: Herbert Gray College, Little Church Street, Rugby CV21 3AP (tel: 01788 573241). They will provide you with a local contact or visit www.relate.org.uk.

BASRT can be contacted on 0208 5432707 or info@basrt.org.uk. www.basrt.org.uk

Further reading
Relate Client Survey January-March 2002 by Jane Roy, available from Relate Central Office.

Reference
[1]Livintoff, S. Relate Guide to Sex in Loving Relationships. Vermilion (£7.99).

5

sex and the menopause

'When you have gone through the menopause you think that sex isn't a part of life anymore — I sometimes think an older gentleman would take a younger partner because of it. Not having sex . . . makes you feel like less of a person . I've never really considered myself as getting old and now I can see different things happening to my body. The sex is not as often as it used to be, so when we do I use a lubricant. After the lubrication and penetration comes the dryness — it's not a comfortable feeling.'
Janet, aged 54.

At the menopause it may be vital to re-think your sex life and how you approach and view sex in order to find a new sexual balance for the next stage of life, which may offer another 30 years of good health. To overcome sexual problems in the period leading up to, during and after the menopause, couples may need to reassess their sexual relationship, taking into account all the ongoing physical and psychological changes.

Part of the assessment may be sexual style, technique and what you both want from the sexual relationship. Rather than allowing sex to 'go on as before' some radical rethinking may have to be done. But it is not easy, especially if sex has become a 'habit' and a painful one at that. It takes real effort and determination and may possibly need the assistance of a therapist to help see you through.

Relationship problems are common at the time of the menopause. A survey in Italy among 175 women taking HRT found that 27% worried about their sex life and of these 79% experienced a loss of libido and 63% a loss of energy. Some 75% of women involved were concerned their partner would lose affection for them. The *Organon Sexuality and Well*

Being Survey in women over 50 published in 2002 involved 1,802 telephone interviews with women aged between 50 and 60 in six European countries and found that:
- 20% had experienced vaginal pain or discomfort during sex
- 60% of these women had subsequently suffered a reduced sex drive.
- 78% of them related their complaints to the menopause although 27% felt it was a consequence of growing older.

The survey revealed that vaginal complaints during sex have a significant effect on women's feelings of self-worth and their enjoyment of life.
- 53% agreed the problems made them feel older
- 59% said their symptoms put them off sex
- 48% said their symptoms sometimes made them feel unhappy
- 42% have sought treatment for vaginal complaints
- 67% who had received treatment had been prescribed lubricants and creams, 25% HRT and 11% natural remedies.

The results showed that sexuality remained important to women in this age group and 80% say that it is very important to maintain a satisfying sex life.
The survey found that:

EFFECTS OF AGEING

Chicago-based Prof. Edward Laumann – whose work has provided the baseline figure of 43% of American women having a sexual problem at some time in the previous 12 months – has discovered that physical factors of ageing do not appear to consistently influence the likelihood of sexual dysfunction.
New work published in 2002 looked at the problems of a lack of interest in sex; an inability to achieve orgasm; physical pain during intercourse; not finding sex pleasurable and lubrication difficulties.
'Social and psychological factors appear to have a much greater impact (than ageing)' he reported in a study conducted by lead researchers from America, Italy, Canada, Brazil and the UK in 30 countries.
There is one solitary area, which does show a link to age – that is 'trouble lubricating'- with 50- to 64-year-olds and 65- to 80-year-olds being 8% and 6%

more likely to report problems than other age groups.
'We can conclude in general that women's sexual dysfunctions notably expect for lubrication problems, are not consistently linked to age.'
One interesting point the researchers observed was that an inability to have an orgasm seems to be a 'Northern European age-linked effect.'
Things that have the greatest impact on women's sexual function appear to be adverse life experiences such as bereavement, divorce, financial problems, and troubled marriages. The findings are in sharp contrast to studies on ED. Strong ageing effects were demonstrated in all countries except one.

The impact of biological ageing effects on the reporting of sexual dysfunctions in women aged 40-80 years: results of an international survey by Edward Laumann et al (see page 19).

- 29% are having sex five times a month
- 18% once a month or less.

But 53% said they had become less interested in sex in the last five years – and this number directly related to the number of menopausal symptoms they had experienced.

When it comes to reduced sex drive, 32% of this population said they had suffered this more in recent years than at any other time in their life. 53% agreed it made them feel older and 35% of them said it sometimes made them feel unhappy.

New research also suggests that women are more likely to experience hypoactive sexual desire disorder after surgical menopause – which occurs when the womb and ovaries are removed – than those who go through the menopause naturally.

A survey of 2,467 European women aged 20 to 70 years, published in the *Journal of Sexual Medicine* in 2006, showed that a greater proportion of surgically menopausal women had low sexual desire compared with pre-menopausal or naturally menopausal women.

A dry vagina is the most common sexual complaints among postmenopausal women, which is physiologically attributed to falling levels of oestrogen. But Dr Ellen Lang, a psychologist at the Department of Clinical Psychology at the University of Amsterdam, says hormones alone may not be the cause. A dry vagina could also signal a problem with sexual arousal and stimulation in some women, which may need a quite different and more natural approach to rectify.

After years in the same sexual relationship sex may have become boring and predictable – and research has confirmed that this situation can kill passion, effectively damaging a woman's ability to become aroused. Some women welcome the menopause as an excuse to cry off having sex with their partners. But with a more imaginative approach to sex, things might improve – if that is what both partners wish. And some extra help through diet or hormonal treatment might encourage sexual response even more.

According to Dr Alessandra Graziottin[1], head of the Female Medical Sexology and Gynaecology Centre in Milan, the idea of older people having a sexual relationship is something of a taboo in our youth-orientated culture. 'Many cultural and emotional biases still prevent many – from lay people to skilled professionals – considering sexuality as a life-long pleasure and a right of the same importance it has in younger subjects.'

Although all the surveys indicate that sex remains important until our 70s and even 80s, doctors rarely raise the topic at consultations with menopausal women.

Does sex change as you get older?

It's not true that sex tends to be something that can only be enjoyed by young people. Sex can be enjoyed as we get older and be just as emotionally satisfying as earlier in life.

The ageing process involves many normal physical changes some of which do affect the sexual response – but sex can and should be more than a focus on the genital aspects. Although sexual function may be different from that of a younger couple: it does not mean it has to be any less pleasurable. Often couples can find new ways to stimulate each other – communication and discussion between partners is important for fulfilling sex to be maintained into later life.

Some women find they take longer to become aroused and this is normal; discussing this with your partner may help him to understand and adapt.

Sexuality is a complex business, and involves the whole 'self' – feelings about yourself as a person, and the functioning of the body, self-esteem, even how you perceive relationships with other people around you. Sometimes a woman's belief in herself as a sexual being is tied to being fertile – an attitude that may change after the menopause.

Looking for love as a widow.

Some women feel guilty even treacherous, if they have lost a loved one but still crave an emotional attachment with a partner.

You may feel awkward and embarrassed and these are normal feelings especially if your partner had a long illness. It will help to talk through these feelings with a counsellor (Try the British Association of Sex and Relationship Therapists). Cruse Bereavement Care provides counselling, advice and social contacts and can be contacted on **020 8939 9530**. Or visit **www.crusebereavementcare.org.uk** or write to **Cruse Bereavement Care, Unit 0.1, 1 Victoria Villas, Richmond, Surrey, TW9 2GW** .

Having sex again after a partner succeeds with Viagra

Some women may have had a break of some years because of a partner's impotence. Professor Annie Potts of the University of Canterbury in Christchurch, New Zealand was the senior researcher on a three-year project investigating the social impact of Viagra. She presented the findings to a conference in Montreal in 2005.

'The use of Viagra can cause tension and conflict in some relationships,' she said. 'Sexual rejuvenation by Viagra can actually precipitate sudden and unwelcome changes, especially if partners had in various ways adjusted to sexual change due to erectile difficulties.'

Key effects of Viagra use by male partners that women in the study found stressful included changes in frequency, duration, and mode of sex, overt and subtle pressures to have sex, tensions and conflicts within relationships, real and imagined infidelities, pressure to maintain a 'youthful' sexuality, and concern for the health of the partner using the drug.

'Men don't want to "waste" a tablet,' said Professor Potts. 'Many women say they put up with sex for the sake of their partner.'

Products and treatments may help to resume the relationship. But this can be a problem especially if the vagina and clitoris feel sore after resumed sexual contact. The answer can be plenty of additional lubrication and taking your time rather than rushing into full penetration.

Discussing sexuality in mid-life or after can be difficult. But remember: sex is normal after middle age and can be an all important part of feelings of well being.

Particular problems of the menopause affecting sexual arousal

- insomnia
- anxiety
- stress
- reduced ability to fantasise and instigate
- mental arousal
- aversion to physical contact
- numbing or tingling sensations
- self-image; loss of fertility, wrinkles, weight gain and possible reduction in breast size and loss of pubic hair due to androgen depletion

These may be compounded by external problems such as
- health
- retirement prospects
- coping with an unfaithful partner
- depression
- physiological changes

The most important change at the menopause is the reduction in levels of oestrogen circulating within the body. But there is also much more awareness now of falling levels of testosterone and how this may have far greater an influence upon older woman's sex drive and response (see *chapter eight – testosterone*).

Before the menopause, the ovaries produce significant amounts of oestrogen as a result of the action of FSH, the follicle-stimulating hormone secreted by the pituitary gland. As the menopause approaches, the ovaries become more resistant to the stimulating effect of FSH and oestrogen production falls.

Your body will undergo some radical changes following the drop in oestrogen: in the genital region vaginas shorten and narrow, there is a loss of fat from the labia majora and labia minora and a reduction in the rate of blood flow to the vaginal tissues, the urethra and the base of the bladder. Vaginal lubrication through the cells of the vaginal wall is an oestrogen-dependent process and although this signal of arousal will still happen it may take longer – just as it can take longer for an older man to get an erection. These changes have long been pinpointed as the reason why menopausal women experience painful sex. But there are added factors: for example, your sense of smell and touch may be altered which can influence how you respond to a sexual partner. You may find that the vaginal area and breasts become less sensitive to touch and orgasm may take longer.

Psychological influences

Research in Holland suggests that not all women who experience physiological changes as a result of the menopause complain of vaginal dryness, pain on intercourse or lack of sexual desire and arousal.

In fact, older women can lubricate almost as well as young women – the key is they may take a little longer. There are many reports of older women in their 70s enjoying sex with their partners without problems.

Dr Laan says in some cases there may be other more fundamental and psychological factors which cause a dry vagina and pain on intercourse. Lubrication is one key element in a woman's enjoyment of sex: without it intercourse can be painful and induce a lasting burning sensation. For good lubrication there must be good sexual stimulation, she says. And that, it seems, is the bottom line. If you are discontented with your partner and don't find him sexually arousing then it may take far longer to become lubricated enough to enjoy pain-free sex. A vicious cycle then develops: you may want to avoid sex altogether and give your partner the cold shoulder.

The good news is that research suggests that new or different types of stimulation will increase the female sexual response in an older woman who is oestrogen deficient. How you might able to apply this in order to enhance your own arousal is explained later in the chapter.

Dr Laan's research has shown that:

- between 5 and 15% of young women also suffer from moderate to severe vaginal dryness – so the problem is not necessarily wholly linked to reduced levels of oestrogen
- women on HRT do not always complain of less vaginal dryness
- women over 50 can lubricate just as well as a younger woman – with the right stimulation

Oestrogen will keep the vagina walls thick and moist, she says, but reduced levels of oestrogen causing a change in the vaginal walls may only accentuate the problem of a lack of arousal (expressed as a dry vagina 'symptom') rather than being the root cause of the problem. 'It may be that an older woman has to try harder or be given more help to be sexually stimulated but it may not be directly linked to falling levels of oestrogen. A younger women may have the advantage of a vaginal wall which is in tip-top condition, but this doesn't mean it is impossible for an older woman.'

These are important findings[2], she says, because it gives an older woman 'permission' to seek out the right sexual stimulation that meets her needs, which may have changed from when she was a young woman and may have changed from what was desired at the start of her long-term relationship with a partner.

'In conclusion it seems that complaints of vaginal dryness and dyspareunia shouldn't be attributed to oestrogen-related vaginal atrophy associated with the menopause. Rather, vaginal dryness and painful intercourse seem to reflect sexual arousal problems.'

More should be done to focus on the different ways in which a woman becomes aroused, advises Dr Laan. This does not necessarily involve laying the responsibility for good sex at the partner's door, although there is no doubt that partners should be aware of a potential problem and help to find new ways to enjoy sex. But she believes more could also be done to investigate biologically what turns women on and how the brain functions in sexual arousal – and whether there are changes as we age.

Supporting this theory is research in Italy which suggests that a new partner may contribute to an increase in libido, satisfaction, and orgasm in post-menopausal women. But if that is not on the agenda, spicing up your own love life with your partner has to be the next best thing.

Couples may need to:

- use more foreplay. Women over 50 do lubricate in response to sexual stimulation, it just may take a little longer
- use extra stimulants such as books or films
- change the ritual of lovemaking: try making love at different times of the day rather than just before bed when you may feel exhausted. Try to pinpoint when you feel most alert: maybe the mornings or the afternoon followed by a nap
- be aware of all the problems which the menopause can cause physically and sexually. For example, the partners of women with touch impairment need to know that affected women are not shunning them physically but that they need help to overcome a very real and painful problem. (You may benefit from HRT at a cellular level but it may not work on your arousal problem)
- find ways to make sex more interesting – regular sex may reduce vaginal deterioration. Men need to take into account their partner's changing needs and not just assume the same pattern and routine expecting responses to be the same as they were. Slow and steady may be an option rather than the dynamic and thrusting approach
- find more comfortable positions and ways for lovemaking. Try instilling a calm atmosphere with dimmed lights or drawn curtains
- introduce some excitement or 'romance'. Women need to be emotionally happy for good sex. Generally, unhappy women have unhappy sex lives. Intimacy is very important and partners may wish to enjoy a closeness without pressure of penetrative sex at every intimate moment.

- be aware of changing circumstances such as children growing up and leaving home and the impact on stress or ill-health upon a woman's sexual function
- make an effort to show affection in the form of holding hands, being close and being tender towards each other

More causes of vaginal dryness

- stress
- excessive douching
- chemotherapy or radiotherapy in the pelvic region

TRY:

- oestrogen creams applied locally (with the advice of a doctor) may help improve the condition of the lining of the womb
- KY-jelly is a faithful standby to lubricate the vagina and is now available as a liquid
- ReplensMD is a special moisturiser for the vagina which only needs to be applied three times a week. The gel consist of polycarbophil, a polymer that retains up to 60 times its own weight in moisture. Because of its special delivery system the gel adheres to the vaginal walls and the moisture contained within it diffuses into vaginal cells. ReplensMD is available from chemists or buy online at **www.anglianpharma.co.uk**
- use moisturisers and gels during foreplay and encourage your partner to indulge in longer foreplay. Spread the lubricant generously over the labia, clitoris, P-spot, and into the vagina as well as on your partner's penis
- be imaginative with sexual foreplay: a gentle massage with sensuous aromatherapy oils, such as sandalwood, might help

'Sex is very important – the problem is I don't have the desire for it anymore,'
– Anna, aged 59.

'I've never really felt he knows truly how to get me to come to climax or arousal. Until recently we haven't been able to have intercourse but have had sexual play. I had my first vaginal repair five years ago having had problems for three years – pain and dryness which has resulted in no sexual intercourse. He had to use a lubricant which took away the spontaneity – and now he can't hold an erection so we are dealing with an ego thing for him,'
– Amy, aged 41.

'After the menopause I had vaginal atrophy, there was no lubrication. I still wanted to have sex because I love him and it's part of our relationship but then it was bleeding and uncomfortable for several days. There was itching and burning – I didn't want to tell him this because he would have shied away from me a little because it would hurt me. So, I didn't

initiate sex because of it. At this stage in my life I could take it or leave it – you need touching and things as you get older, the holding, the sharing of things is important. Over the last seven or eight years we've got a lot closer – we've been married 37 years. If it was just me I'd probably be happy with my life just the way it is but because I also have to consider my partner, it has more meaning,'
– Angela, aged 59.

Other sexual problems of the menopause
TOUCH IMPAIRMENT
As many as 20% of menopausal women experience such skin sensitivity after the menopause that even a partner's gentle loving touch is painful. These levels of pain mean that sex is never pleasurable and can become a burden. It can put a strain on a previously loving relationship – it's desperately hard for a woman to admit that she feels pain when her husband, children or grandchildren hold or touch her or that she cannot even bear the touch of clothes upon her skin. This problem has received little attention or medical acknowledgment but it is a distressing condition which may diminish a woman's sexual desire – because the thought of that painful contact is almost too much to contemplate.

Touch impairment is caused by the changing levels of oestrogen at the menopause which affect the nerves. And it may be linked to another common but largely untalked about problem affecting a loss of sensation or feeling of pain in the clitoris. Affected women describe their clitoris as having gone numb or feel that it is 'dead' and unresponsive. One survey suggests one in five menopausal women experience this problem which may be caused by acute nerve impairment as a result of damaged nerves, or reduced blood flow to the genital area.

Loss of smell and taste
Falling oestrogen levels can affect the sense of smell by as much as 38% after the menopause. Smell can influence libido, reducing the intensity of sexual desire or arousal and affect the ability to detect pheromones which are excreted from the sweat and sebaceous glands of sexual partners. It can also influence the sense of taste and the production of saliva leading to mouth dryness which may influence how you feel about kissing.

Skin problems
The menopause can mean thinning skin, reduced collagen content and a reduction in sebum and release of pheromones. Your skin is one of your sensual organs: if it feels 'different' or thinner it can influence how you view yourself in terms of a sexual partner.

Urinary problems
Something like 60% of menopausal women experience urinary problems – and they do

affect your sex life. Diminishing oestrogen levels affect the tissues around the base of the bladder and urethra and cause leakage at embarrassing moments. This problem during sex is particularly off-putting, and can be a cause of desire disorders. In a series of 201 women referred to a urodynamic clinic for assessment of urinary symptoms most patients said they avoided sexual intercourse and two-thirds directly attributed sexual avoidance to their urinary problems.

Self-image

The transition from fertile to menopausal woman can affect self-perception and self-image, reflecting on your feelings of femininity and sexuality. You may feel 'defeminised' around the time of the menopause contemplating life as an older woman – there is the looming prospect of wrinkles, drier hair and skin, loss of pubic hair and possibly a reduction in breast size, unless you put on weight. (Around the menopause it is common for women to put on weight – maybe up to half a stone. It is a natural way of helping us cope with falling oestrogen levels as we can store oestrogen in fat cells helping us through the withdrawal).

If you feel fat, bad about yourself, or mourn the loss of your fertile years – which may coincide with the blossoming of a teenage daughter into a vital, beautiful, and

---

CASE STUDY

Sally's story

Sally went through the menopause at the age of 40 – she experienced frequent hot flushes and night time sweats – and for the first time in her marriage had to resort to artificial vaginal lubrication. She had always enjoyed making love with her husband and being caressed. But 10 years after the onset of the menopause, she began to notice she felt 'on edge' when her husband touched her, although she still wanted to make love with him. At first her skin felt over-sensitive to the touch – but soon her husband's caresses actually felt painful. It became so severe that she soon found she was being put off sex.

Sally first went to her GP with her symptoms – and was referred to a sex therapist. The therapist suggested Sally and her husband try a course of sensate focus – which proved totally unsuccessful. During therapy, Sally's childhood and teenage sexual development were explored and Sally soon gave up. It was simply not working and it seemed to her irrelevant. Sally was referred to a sex therapy clinic – where it was quickly discovered that she was suffering marked changes around her vagina and vulva – and she was immediately put onto HRT. Eight weeks later she noticed an improvement in her pain problem, and by 12 weeks she was again enjoying her husband's touch. She says she is now feeling better than ever and enjoying a full sex life once again.

Prof. Alan Riley[6] who treated Sally says: 'Sally developed a disturbance in her perception of touch which led her to withdrawing from physical contact with her husband. This was diagnosed by the therapist as a sexual phobic aversion. Had this been the correct diagnosis, it was inappropriate for the therapist to embark upon sensate focus.' Sally was oestrogen-deficient and this was evident from the atrophic changes seen in the vulva and vagina. This case illustrates that post-menopausal women with touch impairment can benefit from HRT.

fertile woman – these feelings can directly affect sexual functioning. Add to this the loss of certain 'extras' such as sensitivity of touch and smell and it is understandable why a whole new approach to your life – and your sex life – might be in order. By taking an interest in yourself as an older, wiser woman, taking up exercise which has been shown to improve sexual functioning, and looking at the positives in your life can, in the long-term, help to turn things around.

During this time of life you may have lost reproductive organs (through hysterectomy), body parts (through mastectomy) or had cancer treatment. All these issues can influence our image of ourselves as sexual beings: negative images will affect our sexual performance. Special help through professional advisers may bolster self-image and esteem and lead to greater understanding that it is acceptance of ourselves and being at peace with our inner selves, which will lead to greater fulfillment.

A positive self-image is linked to greater feelings of well-being and health and can influence a more positive outlook on life with better adjustment to growing older and less depression.

Drugs for menopausal women

New drugs will be aimed at older menopausal women initially. It is a safer bet for the manufacturers because menopausal women don't have babies, therefore reducing the risk of testing the drug on women who may get pregnant during trials. By increasing the blood flow to the clitoris and other genital tissue in response to sensitive sexual stimulation it may be possible to improve orgasm in post-menopausal women. Studies carried out in 1980 showed that after the menopause, blood flow to the clitoris and labia drops.

If a drug is found to improve blood flow, then it may contribute to a restoration of sexual desire and enjoyment in women who find sex painful and difficult. But if Dr Laan is correct then medication for women could only work once the problem of adequate sexual stimulation is addressed.

Preliminary studies on Viagra indicated improved lubrication in a group of post-menopausal women after taking the drug, however trials of the drug have now been suspended. Similar reports for another vasoactive agent – phentolamine – found a 'mild positive effect' among six menopausal women with lubrication difficulties. They all received a single 40mg dose of the drug and 20 minutes later watched an erotic film. There was a slight increase in the rate of vaginal blood flow which lasted for about 15 minutes (women taking a placebo drug showed a lower rate of arousal which lasted for less time).

However, pharmaceutical companies are now largely concentrating their efforts on testosterone treatments for menopausal women. BioSante is testing a new product, LibiGel – a testosterone gel – designed to be used daily for the treatment of FSD. Volunteers in Phase II clinical trials reported a 238% increase in the total number of satisfying sexual events. Phase III trials had just started at the time of writing.

In 2004, Phase III trials showed that Procter & Gamble's testosterone patch, Intrinsa, significantly increased satisfying sexual activity and sexual desire in menopausal women with HSDD and who previously had both ovaries removed. The patch is now available in the UK.

According to research from America older women don't have as many sexual problems as younger women – apart from vaginal dryness. Too many attempts at sex when it is painful can turn into a psychological problem and lead on to an aversion to sex. If you can't communicate well with your partner this may well be misinterpreted as a lack of interest and lead to a deterioration in your relationship.

With the right help to overcome this problem and maybe the addressing of problems of sexual stimulation by means of inventive foreplay or different lovemaking techniques and some self-help measures, there is no reason why women can't go on having orgasms and enjoying sex well into their 70s and 80s – just like men – if the desire or drive is there to do so. There are some 13 million women over the age of 40 in the UK and it is estimated that one in four women feel the need to try HRT because of symptoms of the menopause. Many women over 50 complain that sex is painful, off-putting and unpleasurable – and blame the menopause for this problem and are encouraged to try HRT. But is this really the answer?

HRT is often promoted by GPs as the menopausal woman's universal panacea – to fight osteoporosis and reduce the other problematic consequences of the menopause such as hot flushes and insomnia – and loss of libido.

One variety – Livial, is said to have a positive impact in postmenopausal women who suffer a loss of desire. It contains tibolone, a synthetic compound with weak levels of oestrogen, progesterone and androgen. It provides a bleed-free form of HRT and trials suggest that it improves sexual function for some women (see *chapter seven – treatments*). Dr Laan undertook a trial[3] involving 38 postmenopausal women, with an average age of 54, who received 2.5mg of tibolone a day for three months. They had all reported sex problems after the menopause: on average less sexual satisfaction, arousal, lubrication, although there were no changes in orgasm or pain.

Thirty women (79%) reported an increase in sexual problems after the menopause. Dr Laan measured their responses in two ways: during erotic fantasy sessions and watching erotic films.

She found that after treatment the women all showed an improvement in vaginal blood flow levels – probably due to the oestrogen content of the HRT product. During self-induced fantasy sessions there was a slight increase, but not much improvement during the film sessions.

Dr Laan suggests this may mean women – and men – can be stimulated in different ways, using different brain pathways. Most of the women in the trial using tibolone reported improved sexual function. Improvements on libido and mood have also been found in trials of tibolone in Australia by the Jean Hailes Foundation and the

Department of Obstetrics and Gynaecology in Vienna, Austria.

Many women have anecdotally claimed that HRT can restore their sex lives almost miraculously but research suggests that this effect can wear off after a couple of years. There is some evidence in medical literature to support the idea that HRT can boost sexual desire and that it has a vasoactive effect and enhances blood flow. However, the probability is that HRT or oestrogen replacement has an indirect effect upon libido by helping relieve some of the more distressing or uncomfortable symptoms of menopause.

The effect may be only temporary because it is linked with an improvement in the physical problems of a dry vagina.

The survey[1] by Italian sexologist Dr Grazziotin found that 41% of women felt HRT improved their physical relationship with their partner.

Considerations

The Pennell Initiative has drawn up a detailed report[4] on women's health and says that there are philosophical reasons to be considered before starting hormone replacement therapy. There is a fear that the menopause is becoming 'over-medicalised' and treated as a condition rather than a normal life event.

Before embarking on HRT or ART (Androgen Replacement Therapy), which is available in a few specialist clinics as a testosterone implant, you will have to weigh up the pros and cons for your health. Notably for HRT . . .

- side effects
- fear of increased risk of ovarian or breast cancer
- In 2005, Cancer Research UK's Million Women study found that women who were having HRT at the time of the study were more likely develop breast cancer and die from it that those who had never used HRT. Incidence was significantly increased for users of preparations containing oestrogen only, oestrogen-progestagen and tibolone. However, when the treatment is stopped the risk is reduced and disappears after about five years. The study concluded that use of HRT by women aged 50-64 years in the UK over the past decade has resulted in an estimated 20,000 extra breast cancers, with 15,000 of these associated with oestrogen-progestagen.
- coming to terms with taking a drug over a long period of time . . and for ART
- risk of masculinisation if testosterone levels are too high
- possible increase in cholesterol levels in susceptible post-menopausal women (an issue still being studied). This could heighten the risk of heart disease.

The Pennell Initiative recommends that at around the age of 50 women might benefit from a health and lifestyle consultation to discuss 'all aspects of the menopause and long-term health'. The Initiative says: 'It is important that women and the men in their lives have information about the menopause and its possible implications for them.'

HRT is **not recommended** for women with a history of:
- cancer of the breast, genital tract or other oestrogen-dependent cancers
- vaginal bleeding
- endometriosis
- thrombosis
- cardiac, liver or kidney disease
- migraine (sufferers may experience a recurrence of the problem after taking HRT)
- MS
- fibroids

but HRT and ART **may be useful** for women
- who have had an early menopause
- who have had a surgical menopause – i.e. a hysterectomy and removal of the ovaries before the natural menopause and complain of loss of sexual desire or arousal
- those at increased risk of osteoporosis

The possible risks of HRT are:
- endometrial cancer
- breast cancer – there have been more than 40 studies but no obviously consistent results: some show an increased risk when HRT is used for five years or more
- thrombosis – there may be a slight increase in the risk of thrombosis during the first year of using HRT – it may be particularly high among women with a family history of this problem.

Phytoestrogens
These components of certain common foods, (also known generically as isoflavones) are powerful natural chemicals which have a marked, similar structure to oestrogen but are far less potent. Doctors are expressing some interest but say more research is needed to be confident of their benefits as an alternative to HRT. Phytoestrogens are present in beans and pulses but a herb called red clover (now sold as a food supplement) and soya products contain the highest concentrations.

Research indicates they have the power to block the uptake of excess oestrogen in the body and even raise low levels where necessary and it seems they mimic oestrogen's role in the body competing successfully for receptor sites at the entrance to cells. There is medical interest in their ability to alleviate many common diseases affecting women such as breast cancer, osteoporosis, and heart disease.

The effect on vaginal dryness has been more difficult to prove: few studies have shown a significant impact upon vaginal wall improvement. However, they might help contribute to an overall sense of well-being.

Genistein

Genistein is the most extensively studied phytoestrogen and is found only in soya – it was identified as a plant oestrogen in 1966. According to Maryon Stewart writing in her book, *The Phyto Factor*[5], genistein has a role in reducing oestrogen withdrawal symptoms at the menopause 'including hot flushes, night sweats, dry vagina and insomnia'.

In 1990, a body of Australian researchers found that a group of women going through the menopause who regularly consumed food and drink containing naturally occurring oestrogen brought about the same improved changes to the lining of their vagina as women taking HRT.

In 1992, a study in *The Lancet* concluded that Japanese women do not experience symptoms of the menopause because their diet is rich in plant oestrogens. (For example, the incidence of hot flushes in menopausal women in Europe is between 70 and 80%, 57% in Malaysia and just 18% in China.) Soya is at the centre of the GM (genetically modified) scare – for pure untainted soya, check health food stores and read the labels.

Foods rich in phytoestrogens which may help the symptoms of menopause are:

- golden linseeds which can be sprinkled over cereal in the mornings
- red clover which can be taken as a food supplement
- soya products such as soya milk, soya yoghurt, beans, flour and even cream or cheese
- miso, which is a fermented soya bean paste
- tofu – a textured vegetarian protein used as a meat substitute found in health food stores
- chick peas, lentils, mung beans and aduki beans
- Burgen bread, a soya and linseed loaf available at most big supermarkets

Progesterone cream

Californian doctor and writer Dr John Lee has argued for many years that the falling levels of progesterone rather than oestrogen after the menopause cause so many of the symptoms including loss of libido. He manufactures a natural progesterone cream derived from yams, and like phytoestrogens it mimics progesterone in the body. Trials into the effectiveness of progesterone cream have been staged at the

GUIDELINES TO A HEALTHY MENOPAUSE

- stop smoking
- eat a healthy diet rich in fruit and vegetables
- try to maintain a healthy weight
- increase your exercise – particularly weight-bearing exercise such as walking
- have your blood pressure checked
- control high cholesterol levels

Chelsea and Westminster Hospital. Volunteers applied progesterone cream every day for 48 weeks. Plasma levels of progesterone increased after 12 weeks, however there was no further evidence of accumulation of progesterone in the remaining weeks. Researchers say that further study is needed to assess the safety and efficacy of this treatment. Progesterone cream is only available on prescription.

St. John's Wort

Hypericum is proving to be a very useful herb for treating depression, but a trial in Germany also suggests it can revive sexual interest. A study of 11 women in Germany who experienced a loss of desire at the time of the menopause were given a 12-week course of the herb. Some 60% reported they had regained their libido whilst 80% generally felt better.

The WNAS recommend taking 900mgs of hypericum for three months to test the effects.

(**Note:** St John's Wort should not be taken with other anti-depressants or during pregnancy or when breast-feeding. Check with your doctor first if you are taking medication).

Sensual exercises for older couples

There is still an element of resistance in society to the idea of older couples having sex – and enjoying it. But it is important to recognise that sexuality is natural and normal and can be highly erotic and enjoyable at an older age – although there can be more to sexuality than vaginal intercourse.

There are plenty of other ways to improve and nurture intimacy and sexual feelings. These can range from holding hands, hugging, caressing or kissing closely to masturbation and oral sex, and can bring about a sense of closeness even when sex is difficult or painful. Touching, smelling, hearing and visual sensations are all part of sexuality and can be used to help improve feelings of sexual desire.

If you are having difficulty with night sweats and insomnia it might help take pressure off by having one bed for your intimate times and a single bed for sleeping. But strengthening your sexuality through contact is important even when full intercourse is not desirable.

If your children have left home, think about other times for lovemaking: traditionally you may have made love just before bedtime. But as you get older or go through the menopause you may feel exhausted at this time: sex is best when you are relaxed and alert. Try to find some other time during the day. The early afternoon may be great. The message is: ring the changes, it may just help to reawaken your sexual interest.

Talking about fantasies and desires might also help (see *chapter twelve – fantasy and lovemaking techniques*) but what is all important is communicating to your partner your needs and desires. Rather than shrugging your partner off, talk about the changes that are happening and different ways in which you can express affection for each other.

Spend plenty of time on foreplay, holding, stroking and caressing each other: slowly but surely rather than 'quickie' sex may suit you. If you feel a loss of attraction for your partner it may be worth trying psycho-sexual counselling: working out your feelings with a third party can help you and help your partner to understand what might be happening.

Somehow we expect our partners to know telepathically how we are feeling and why, without communicating the facts. If your feelings are out in the open then they can be worked upon, and, hopefully improved.

If you or your partner have a chronic physical complaint or condition consider changing your sexual styles or techniques, or maybe investigate different lovemaking positions.

Talk to your doctor if you are on anti-depressants or medication for hypertension – certain drugs will affect sexual functioning. You may be anxious about your sexual functioning after having a hernia repair, hysterectomy, or surgery for incontinence or womb prolapse.

Bear in mind that exercise will improve general muscle tone and overall health and feelings of well-being. If sex is fun for you both, then it can only be doing you good. Laughter is one of nature's greatest healers.

Love and getting older

Masters and Johnson, the famous sexologists, were the first to suggest that sexuality can robustly continue into old age and many studies have since confirmed their conclusions – with the additional bonus that sexual health is not just a reflection of good health but actively contributes to it.

The importance of sensual and tactile experiences in later life is underlined in a report[4], *Sexuality and the Older Woman*, published in April 2001 by the Pennell Institute. It suggests that sex contributes to a healthy lifestyle post-45 and into old age. 'Sex may be one of several activities that may have a buffering effect against certain illnesses,' it says.

But the report found there was a lack of sensitivity and awareness among health professionals regarding the expression of sexuality in older women. It also stressed how little is known about the long term effects of illness, disability, and being in a relationship on older women and their sexuality.

Chris Vincent, of the Tavistock Marital Studies Institute, and one of the report's authors said: 'Myths and prejudice colour our views of sexuality and ageing. This review seeks to demystify what for many remains a taboo subject. 'It demonstrates that for many older women sexual experience is a key component of a full and healthy life.'

The report confirms: 'Sexual drive and intensity diminishes in later life with the result that other forms of sexual satisfaction become increasingly important. These include autoerotic as well as inter-personal experiences – for example having one's hair washed or wearing nice clothes.'

The report calls for more health professionals to recognise sexual health is important for older women and recommends that because of the importance of sex older women should be referred to specialists on FSD when appropriate.

In her study[1], *Sexuality and the Elderly,* Dr Graziottin suggests that some women can experience 'the life surprise' – the gift of having new loves and partners in old age.

'This rejuvenating experience is emotionally rewarding, but may raise new sexual problems particularly if one or both partners had remained alone for years. Also, in these cases, a caring doctor could be precious in treating the problems that could prevent a satisfying intimacy.'

She reported the case of a woman of 69 who fell in love with a widower aged 73 and attended the clinic to ask 'Doctor, will you help me to be a little bit happy?' She was suffering from vaginismus, reports the doctor, but after behavioural therapy and a course of HRT she went on to experience the first orgasm of her life at the age of 70. Dr Grazziotin said: 'At the five year follow-up they are one of the happiest couples I know.'

How to help yourself

Don't let resentment take over – talk to someone if one partner's needs are not being met by the other and there is a subsequent imbalance in expectations. It is natural for an illness or depression to put you off sex for a while. But don't let it become an issue – there may be a simple answer. New medication may be putting you off sex: your GP may consider altering it.

Remember that older women do need more foreplay to become aroused. Inserting the penis before lubrication may be the cause of pain.

References

[1]Graziottin, A. Sexuality in the Elderly. European Congress on Menopause, ESKA Editions, 1998. 513-520

[2]Hormones and Sexuality post-menopause, *Journal of Psychosomatic Obstetric Gynaecology* 1997. **18**: 126-133,.

[3]Laan. E, *et al.* The effects of tibolone on vaginal blood flow, sexual desire, and arousability in postmenopausal women, Department of Clinical Psychology, University of Amsterdam. Climacteric 2001. **4**: 28-41.

[4]The Pennell Reports, The Pennell Initiative, Health Services Management Unit, University of Manchester, Devonshire House, Precinct Centre, Oxford Road, Manchester M13 9PL (tel 0161 275 2910).

[5]Stewart, M; *The Phyto Factor*, Vermilion.

[6]Riley, A.J. Sexuality and the Menopause. *Sexual and Marital Therapy* 1991 Vol. 6, No. 2.

6

painful sex

Sarah is in her late 20s. Life should be full of promise – but she says she has contemplated suicide. The reason? She cannot have sex. While friends are in loving relationships, she has to look in from the outside. She feels like a loner because she has a rare condition called lichen sclerosus: it is so painful that she is unable to have a sexual relationship with a partner.

It is estimated that 15% of women experience painful sex at some time. (Painful intercourse is called dyspaurenia by doctors.) Women suffering from conditions relating to vulval pain are most often aged between 20 and 45 although women outside this age range can also be affected.

There is now a recognised 'cycle of pain', which starts in the vulva, moving to fear of pain and anticipation of pain during sex, followed by partial avoidance of sexual intimacy, as a protection against pain, to sexual arousal disorder, loss of sexual desire, problems with orgasm, total avoidance of sexual activity and relationship difficulties.

Dr David Nunns, a gynaecologist and chairman of the Vulval Pain Society, says women often don't seek help until they reach the point of sexual avoidance and relationship difficulties. But it is important to try and find some help before it reaches this stage. Many problems are short-lived and can be remedied with treatment coupled with reassurance.

But some women suffer from more prolonged painful conditions that can last for years. There are a host of reasons for these kind of problems, which is why you should try and see a specialist. Deep and burning pain often felt up in the pelvis during sex can be caused by of a lack of lubrication, infection or other problems such as endometriosis.

There may be pain if there is failure of the womb to rise and the vagina to balloon to accommodate the penis, or when there is pelvic inflammatory disease or prolapsed ovaries. External vaginal pain may be caused by a condition called vestibulitis, an inflammatory problem, genital herpes, or an acute infection of the vagina.

There may be sensitivity to contraceptive creams or barrier methods of contraception such as the cap or condoms. Diabetic women are prone to thrush which can cause soreness and irritation. A dermatologist best deals with specific vulval skin conditions such as lichen sclerosus, eczema, and skin inflammation.

Gundi Kiemle, consultant clinical psychologist at the Bolton Centre for Sexual Health, Royal Bolton Hospital, says: 'Sexual dysfunction in women with vulval pain is common, but not inevitable.

'When it occurs it is important for the woman and her partner to be aware that sexual problems can be treated and help is available.

'When sexual problems are ignored the woman may find herself in a position where months or years later her vulval condition has improved with or without treatment but in the meantime she has lost her sexual desire and may even be experiencing more general relationship difficulties, as a result of long term avoidance.'

Common causes of short term or occasional pain

VAGINAL THRUSH

This is caused by an overgrowth of the yeast *Candida albicans*. It's naturally present in the body in up to one-third of women but normally does not cause symptoms or problems. Thrush develops when the yeast overgrows in the vagina – which may be happen after a course of antibiotics, during pregnancy, and if you have diabetes.

Symptoms are vulval itching, soreness and discharge and it can be painful to pass urine, which can irritate the inflamed and sore vulval skin. There may be nothing to see on examination – or there might be redness and swelling of the vulval skin. A GP can confirm thrush with a vaginal swab test and it can be treated with creams, pessaries or tablets. Try over-the-counter remedies such as Canestan and Diflucan.

Recurrent thrush can be a problem for some women and may result in them being put off sex because of soreness and irritation. Symptoms of recurrent thrush can be mistaken for other vulval complaints such as vulvodynia and vulval vestibulitis, so get checked out if you suffer repeatedly.

AFTER HAVING A BABY

Many women complain that sex is painful after having a baby. It might

---

CONDITIONS THAT MAY CAUSE PAINFUL SEX

Eczema
Lichen Planus
Lichen sclerosus
Lichen simplex
Psoriasis
Pemphigus vulgaris
Pemphigoid
Zoon vulvitis
Vulvodynia
Vaginismus
Vestibulitis
Thrush
Genital herpes
Shingles
Hidradenitis suppuravita
Molluscum contagiosum
Tinea
Warts
Chlamydia
Cancer
Vulval lymphangioma
Paget's disease
Bechet's disease.

be that perineal stitches have healed too tightly, or there may be inflammation. Oestrogen levels fall after child-birth, especially if a mother is breast-feeding. This can result in a feeling of vaginal dryness: using extra lubrication may help to overcome this temporary problem.

Some new mothers also experience anxiety about sex and an involuntary spasm in the vaginal muscles at the time of intercourse. 'This may be a guarding response,' explains David Nunns. A woman who experiences this problem will recover with lots of reassurance, and possibly relaxation techniques such as sensate focus which helps partners 'reconnect' without penetrative sex initially. Vaginal dilators may also help. Femmax dilators are available on NHS prescription or through the National Lichen Sclerosus Support Group for £15.00 (including Vat and P&P). For more information visit www.lichensclerosus.org or write to the National Lichen Sclerosus Support Group, PO Box 5830, Lyme Regis, Dorset, DT7 3PT.

Long-term pain
LICHEN SCLEROSUS
This is a poorly recognised and misunderstood condition. Any area of skin can be affected – although most commonly it is the genitals. There is no cure but there is treatment that can offer relief: steroid and soothing aqueous creams.

The cause is not known, but the condition is thought to be an auto immune response and has strong links to thyroid conditions, vitiligo and pernicious anaemia. It is estimated that between 1 in 300 and 1 in 1000 people are affected – but it is not contagious and cannot be transmitted via sex.

KEY SYMPTOMS
- Chronic itching
- The skin may split causing stinging and pain
- Vulval skin will become pale and white in appearance
- Maybe more bouts of thrush

LS is essentially a chronic inflammatory skin disease that affects the vulva – it does not extend into the vagina. Any area of the skin can be affected but most commonly the genital area. It mainly affects adult women. However, it can and does affect women at any age and also men and young children. There is some speculation, as yet unproved, that LS may be genetic.

Symptoms include chronic, intractable itching and soreness of the vulval area. The skin may split, causing stinging and pain. The anal opening can also be affected. The skin will sometimes split and bleed on passing bowel motions, causing discomfort. The vulval skin becomes fragile and pale in appearance. There is increased susceptibility to infection and bouts of thrush. There may be atrophy (shrinking/wasting of the skin) causing the contours of the vulval area to reduce and change in appearance and some women suffer a narrowing of the vaginal opening.

In some cases there may be fusion of the labia minora, the urethra (causing urination difficulties) and of the clitoris, which can become buried. There may be a tendency for the skin to split or tear during sexual intercourse. Many sufferers abstain from sex for long periods of time until symptoms can be brought under control. There is a small risk of cancer estimated at between 3% and 5%.

Diagnosis can be difficult and has been known to take several years. There is a lack of awareness among GPs who often misdiagnose and treat the condition for years as thrush. Some GPs may not have heard of the condition or have ever seen a case in their surgery during the course of their career.

Patients may also be told that their symptoms are being caused by age, hormones, menopause, STDs, vaginitis or psychological reasons. If itching (or any of the other symptoms stated in the previous paragraph) have been present for six months to a year with no improvement, it is advisable to ask for a referral to a gynaecologist or dermatologist. Very often the presence of LS is discovered when a consultation has been sought for another unrelated condition. A skin biopsy should be performed to confirm the presence of LS and rule out any malignancy. This involves taking a small piece of skin from the affected area under local anaesthetic.

Treatment is to relieve the effects of symptoms only but can be very effective. Topical steroid creams/ointments are prescribed and a wide range of preparations is available. Not everyone responds to the same type of steroid preparation and it may be necessary to persevere with various products.

Many women experience quite long remissions in symptoms after treatment but sometimes the symptoms return. Surgery is not a treatment for LS but is sometimes necessary to alleviate the effects of scarring or fusion, or if the vaginal opening has narrowed making intercourse difficult.

VULVAL CARE

The advice from the medical professionals is to avoid the use of all soaps, gels and scented products in the bath and shower as these may contain irritants. Aqueous cream is recommended for cleaning the vulval area. It is inexpensive and easily available and it can also be helpful and soothing for cleaning the anal area.

Aqueous cream kept in the fridge can be helpful to just dab (not rubbed in) an ample amount onto the vulva to give a cooling, soothing effect. Avoid wearing tights, jeans, or tight trousers. Avoid using hard, scratchy flannels for washing the vulva and use your hand to apply the aqueous cream for washing.

Dab the vulval area gently to dry or try using a hairdryer on a cool setting and held well away from the skin. Also avoid washing underwear in biological washing powders, and wash and rinse these items separately from your main wash.

Women with LS may experience a narrowing of the vaginal opening. Some dermatologists say that maintaining regular sexual intercourse will help to prevent the vaginal opening from becoming narrow. If you do not have a sexual partner, maintaining the vaginal opening will be more difficult but regular use of vaginal dilators may help. Always use a good lubricant gel on the dilator before attempting to insert it. Some women report an increase in confidence regarding their sexual ability as a result of using dilators.

PELVIC INFLAMMATORY DISEASE

Chlamydia is the most common form of PID (pelvic inflammatory disease). Women who use intra-uterine contraceptive devices (IUDs) can be at risk from infection and subsequent painful sex. If left untreated, pelvic infections can cause inflammation and adhesions. These may continue to give problems long after the infection itself has settled. The symptoms of PID may flare up when you are run down, and can be hard to treat, although a GP will prescribe antibiotics.

OVARIAN CYSTS

Ovarian cysts, which can show up on a scan or internal examination, can cause painful sex.

Vaginismus

This problem involves the muscles of the pelvic floor, which surrounds the vagina – if the muscles tense up it makes vaginal entry difficult. Some women experience an uncontrolled spasm that effectively cuts off entry to the vagina – they may arch their back as if trying to escape.

A woman who repeatedly suffers from this can inevitably be put off sex, even though their drive may still be intact. There may be a psychological association - possibly linked to a past trauma such as rape or abuse – which triggers this response. The response is said to be a guarding response to pain.

Vaginismus can be treated. Psychosexual counselling may help, along with the use of vaginal dilators. This condition can lead to sexual dysfunction – when sex equals pain there is a reluctance to try again. The pain needs to be resolved but the sufferer may later need extra help to overcome the association between pain and sex.

Ulcers

The same type of ulcers people get in the mouth can also be found on the vulva and this can cause painful sex.

Vulvodynia

This can be the cause of immense and constant pain for some women. It is often described as a burning aching sensation and may be so severe as to prevent some women from sitting down comfortably. It's as if nerve fibres are all switched to 'on' mode causing constant pain. The condition commonly affects women over 40. This kind of pain is best treated with drugs that alter the way nerve fibres send impulses to the spinal cord, giving the sensation of pain. Gabapentin is an anti-convulsive drug used for chronic pain management.

Vaginal lubricants can help during intercourse, Try oatmeal baths, aqueous cream, aloe vera gel, or calendula cream for natural relief from pain. Some women find acupuncture helps.

Vestibulitis

This is an inflammation causing considerable pain around the vagina – the vestibule is the area where the vulva meets the vagina and is extremely sensitive. It contains the Bartholin's glands, which lubricate the vagina. The pain experienced by this condition is very individual – but there is no pain until the area is touched. For some women the pain is present given the lightest touch, others can tolerate intercourse. This is a very real, physical disease and should be diagnosed by a doctor after ruling out infections or other problems.

Treatments range from anaesthetic creams (such as Lignocaine) to pelvic floor physiotherapy and psychosexual counselling. Often there is no known cause – although some women suffer after an attack of thrush. Some women complain of the problem after childbirth and sufferers of interstitial cystitis are another susceptible group.

Unresolved pain

There is a group of women for whom everything appears normal yet who suffer form unexplained pain during sex. Dr Nunns says that around 60% of this group of women

---

SEX AND
VULVAL PAIN

Vulval pain affects sexual functioning. Most sufferers are aged between 20-45 years.
A study of 45 women with vulval vestibulitis syndrome (VVS) carried out in 1992 (Schover *et al*) found that 60 per cent of women complained of vaginismus (involuntary spasm of the pelvic floor muscles surrounding the vagina, effectively making penetration impossible), 57 per cent were unable to achieve orgasm in certain situations, 57 per cent had problems with vaginal lubrication or expansion during sex (the normal changes which usually take place during arousal), 51 per cent had low sexual desire, and 49 per cent also complained of poor sexual communication. Furthermore, six per cent had a complete aversion to sex.

Another study in 1997 compared 105 women with pain during sexual intercourse including 54 with vulval vestibulitis syndrome, to 105 pain-free controls. The VVS sub-group were less sexually active, had less frequent sexual intercourse, lower levels of sexual desire and arousal, and less likelihood of achieving orgasm, either through oral sex or intercourse, compared to the pain-free controls.

may have experienced unresolved sexual abuse in the past. They would be offered psychotherapy. 'It is important for doctors to ask the right questions,' he stresses. 'This is a physical expression of psychological problems. A women may put up a physical barrier to sex if she has unresolved issues. Those barriers need to be broken down.'

Self-help: What can I do to help myself?

Try to banish thoughts and feelings of embarrassment when it comes to problems and pain involving the vulva. The vulva is simply part of the body. Prof. Riley, the UK's first professor of sexual medicine, says: 'We see so many women who have never examined their own vulva – disowning it rather than accepting that part of their bodies. Unless a woman can be encouraged to have a healthy accepting attitude to her vulva she will not recognise early manifestations of vulval disease.'

Self-examination

First, find a private place such as the bathroom or bedroom. Using a mirror try and get a good view of the vulval area by separating the outer lips.

Start at the top – the mons pubis – which is the area above the vagina around the public bone. Then work down checking the clitoris, labia minora, labia majora, perineum and finally the anus.

LOOK FOR:
- Any changes of colour such as whitening or increase in skin pigmentation
- Any thickening of the skin such as warts, lumps or skin tags
- Any ulcers or sores particularly those that don't heal
- Symptoms of persistent itchiness or soreness

If you learn what looks normal for you then you'll quickly realise what is abnormal.

Treatments and investigation
- Antibiotics for chlamydia
- Hormonal treatments for endometriosis
- Laparoscopy – to investigate deep inside the pelvis to see if there are any other reasons for the pain.
- Vaginal dilators. Amielle Vaginal Dilators are an effective aid to treatment of vaginismus, dyspareunia and post radiotherapy adhesions and scarring. Amielle Vaginal Dilators are available as a full set that includes four cones in graduated sizes, a twist and lock handle for ease of insertion, cleaning brush and tube of aqua gel for lubricating the cones. The full set is packaged in a discreet zipped carrying bag. A full set costs £39.95 including VAT. Amielle is available on prescription and can be ordered from the Owen Mumford Medical Shop on freephone 0800 731 6959 or visit **www.mumford.com**.

- Biofeedback may help some women resume sexual intercourse. A study published in the *Journal of Reproductive Medicine*[1] in 1995 involving 33 women with vulval vestibulitis used biofeedback to reduce the spasm, or tension in pelvic floor muscles. After an average of 16 weeks' practice, 22 out of 28 women had resumed sexual intercourse and 17 out of 33 reported pain-free sexual intercourse.
- Sensate focus. (see *chapter four – sex and the mind*)
- Surgery. Removal of the vulval (vulvectomy) has major implications for a woman's sex life. Often the clitoris is removed, although the vagina will usually remain unaffected. Women will be able to have sex but the vulval area will look and feel different. Some feeling may be lost. Discuss the effects with your doctor first.

Other vulval complaints

VULVAL CANCER

Around 700 to 1,000 women a year are diagnosed with vulval cancer which makes it a rare condition. Like all cancers, it can be lethal unless it is treated early.

The Vulval Pain Society have issued a leaflet explaining how women can examine themselves regularly, in the same way they are encouraged to examine their breasts for lumps. The Society recommends examination should be done once a month or any time when you develop vulval itching, or pain, find sex painful, or if you feel lumps or thickening of the skin. Learning to take care of this very special part of your body should be as important to you as making regular breast examinations, they say.

All about the vulva

During the course of a woman's life time, the vulva undergoes many changes, it has to cope with monthly cycles, thrush infections, intercourse without sufficient lubrication, and childbirth. We crush our vulva into tight and unsuitable clothing.

Medically, vulval conditions are considered low profile and low priority. Vulval disorders are still poorly recognised or misdiagnosed by a high percentage of family practitioners, making it extremely important that you recognise the need to be aware and take care of your vulva.

The pain and sex aversion cycle

- Vulval pain
- Fear of pain and anticipation of pain during sex
- Partial avoidance of sexual intimacy and activity (seen as protection again pain)
- Sexual arousal disorder (insufficient or no vaginal expansion and lubrication)
- Loss of sexual desire
- Problems with orgasm
- Total avoidance of sexual activity
- Relationship difficulties

Useful addresses

Vulval Pain Society, PO Box 7804, Nottingham, NG3 5ZQ. www.vulvalpainsociety.org. Information and advice on all vulval diseases, including dietary treatments and explanations of the conditions. They publish *The Vulval Pain Society Handbook*, a comprehensive guide to vulval conditions and self-help measures.

The Thrush Advice Bureau, PO Box 8762, London, SW7 4ZD. Helpline 0207 2855523. www.thrushadvice.co.uk

British Thyroid Foundation, PO Box 97, Clifford, Wetherby, West Yorkshire LS23 6XD. 01423 709707. www.btf-thyroid.org

Vitiligo Society, 125 Kennington Road, London, SE11 6SF. Helpline 0800 0182631. www.vitiligosociety.org

Vulval clinics – where to find them?

Vulval clinics are often all-women teams and include a gynaecologist, skin specialist, doctor and sex therapist. But they are few and far between. Contact the British Society for the Study of Vulval Diseases for a comprehensive list of specialists in your area. Their website is: www.bssvd.org. Or call 01925 662476

References

[1]Glazer, H. I., *et al.* Treatment of vulvar vestibulitis syndrome with electromyographic biofeedback of pelvis floor musculature. *Journal of Reproductive Medicine* 1995. **40** (4): 283-290.

7

trials and tribulations
– new treatments

I f you believe you are suffering from FSD you'll want to know what help is available. Treatments for FSD mainly fall into two distinct groups – drugs delivered in a variety of ways from pills to sprays, patches, and vaginal tablets, to gadgets or specially designed sex toys designed to stimulate or reawaken interest.

There are more than 20 products currently being developed to treat FSD, according to the World Health Organisation, including pills, hormone patches and gels. But to date there is no medication on the market that is licensed for female sexual dysfunction. There are, however, approved drugs that have been found to help, such as some forms of HRT and testosterone implants.

Trials are underway for new medications, and you may want to help test new drugs. This might be possible to organise through your doctor or via interested specialists known to the Sexual Dysfunction Association.

Unless you are one of the women involved in current trials, it is unlikely that any drugs for female impotence will become available in the UK within the next year. Even then it is unlikely they will be able to provide 'instant orgasms'.

Drugs are being tested in three key areas to see if it is possible to:
- improve blood flow which may help women with specific physiological problems
- address a loss of desire with hormonal treatment
- work on centres in the brain that may be linked to sexual functioning – a large UK study is underway involving a drug commonly prescribed for Parkinson's Disease

Although new medications will probably not reach the market place in the very near future, there has been a resurgence of interest in modern vibrators designed for women, by women. These look nothing like the phallic 'rocket' style vibrators: modern vibrators are gently curved and designed more specifically for clitoral stimulation.

Research around the world suggests it is a lack of interest in sex that has been becoming more common over the years. This poses quite a different challenge to the 'mechanical' physiological problem of ED – and that makes finding a medication that works for women more complex. But in the future it may be possible to help women with special problems like arterial disease or diabetes, where an improved blood flow to the vagina and genitals may help the sexual response. We predict that a small range of drugs will come onto the market that will offer some women real hope of an improvement in the way they feel about sex. And just having drugs available will, hopefully, open the doors to more discussion and understanding, more GP awareness, and will help women to feel confident about approaching a doctor or other health professional – or their partner – to discuss their problem.

The drugs

A variety of formulations are being developed by drugs companies such as:

- pills
- nasal sprays
- gels
- creams
- skin patches
- vaginal tablets
- HRT with 'extras'.
- topical oils

Alternatives are:

- herbs
- supplements
- gadgets and stimulation devices
- surgery

Pills

VIAGRA

Viagra was first developed as a treatment for heart disease. This phosphodiesterase PDE5 inhibitor displayed little effect on the cardiovascular system but men with ED found an unexpected improvement in erectile performance.

Viagra works by increasing the effects of the body chemical nitric oxide, which is responsible for regulating the flow of blood to the genitals. This increased blood flow makes erections in men easier. Viagra became an overnight 'blockbuster' drug in March 1998, setting records with millions of dollars' worth of sales in its first two months on the market.

It is estimated that nine of the blue diamond shaped tablets are now dispensed every second, and that more than 23 million men have had prescriptions written. Pfizer reported sales of $1.65bn in 2005. They hoped to produce another blockbuster with Viagra for women. But in 2004, after eight years of tests involving 3,000 women, Pfizer abandoned efforts to prove that the drug works for females too.

The majority of women tested in clinical trials were those who had passed the menopause and others who had hysterectomies, although one trial in Italy involved women in their 20s and 30s, many of whom said they had sex more often and had more sexual fantasies. Dr Jennifer Berman announced findings of a study involving 202 women with sexual arousal problems at the International Society for the Study of Women's Sexual Health in Vancouver in October 2002. Fifty two of these women were post menopausal, while 150 had hysterectomies. They were given either Viagra or a dummy drug for 12 weeks and asked to record changes in their love lives. More patients reported increased sensation and satisfaction with Viagra than the placebo – 57 per cent reported improved sensation during intercourse, although so did 44 per cent using the dummy drug.

It was found that the ability to orgasm was increased among a substantial number of women, and the effect was felt best in those who wanted sex but did not usually enjoy it. Pfizer said they were cautiously optimistic about 'pink Viagra' but a year later announced that they were suspending trials, because of inconclusive data about the drugs efficacy.

'There's a disconnect in many women between genital changes and mental changes,' Dr Mitra Boolel, of Pfizer, said at the time. 'This disconnect does not exist in men. With women, arousal depends on a myriad of factors.'

Dr Joe Feczko, president of worldwide development with the company, added 'FSAD is an emerging area of research and is far more complex than male erectile dysfunction. Diagnosing FSAD involves assessing physical, emotional and relationship factors, and these complex and interdependent factors make measuring a medicine's effect very difficult.'

Pfizer is now concentrating on developing drugs that directly affect a woman's brain chemistry. That is not to say that women will not still try the drug. It is estimated that 17 per cent of women with FSD in America are prescribed Viagra even though it has not been licensed for women.

Other similar drugs

Drug companies are investigating whether two other PDE5 antagonists called vardenafil (being looked at by Bayer) and tadalafil (Lilly-ICOS) may work in the same way.

ANTIDEPRESSANTS

- Wellbutrin (buproprion) is an antidepressant which may also help to improve sexual drive. One trial suggested that as many as 29% of women reported improved feelings of sexual desire and in another small trial, four out of 20 women with orgasm problems showed an increase in sexual desire after nine weeks.

At least a third of people who take the class of antidepressants which includes Prozac have problems with sexual arousal. But so far no new drug has become available.

Patches, gels, creams and oils

INTRINSA AND TOSTRELLE – TESTOSTERONE (ANDROGEN) THERAPIES

Sex hormones or, more specifically, certain component parts play a vital part in arousal and excitement. They act on sensory organs and can determine libido – the motivational force for sex. The clitoris, labia and nipples are constructed of androgen-dependent tissues. Although testosterone is generally considered to be a male hormone it is produced by the ovaries in women and is the 'fuel' which triggers the sex drive through its stimulating action upon androgen dependent tissues. Women need a certain level of the hormone to maintain proper sexual functioning. (Women who lose their ovaries before the menopause lose about half their natural testosterone.) As we age, levels of testosterone drop, and a shortage or imbalance may explain why some women do not experience sexual feelings (see *chapter eight – testosterone*).

Women in America have woken up to the idea of testosterone patches following an Oprah Winfrey show about the hormone. The main job is convincing women of the safety of the drug and reassuring them they won't suffer from side effects such as hairy faces. Various companies are looking at androgens in different delivery forms – patches, gels and creams – and gathering more evidence about its impact on sexual desire. Women who are given testosterone replacement therapy often report extra benefits such as less fatigue, improved well-being, and higher libido.

Although the Food and Drug Authority in America rejected Procter and Gamble's application for a licence for Intrinsa, the patch has been licensed in Europe. However, Intrinsa is designed to help a very specific group of women and it is only available on prescription in the UK to surgically menopausal women under 60.

The Sexual Dysfunction Association is expecting an increase in calls from women with questions about Intrinsa now that the patch is available. However, Helpline advisor Ilaria Primoni says that very few of women who currently contact the SDA are likely to benefit from the launch.

'Most of the women who contact us don't have gynaecological problems and they're not post-menopausal. They are in their 20s and 30s and have arousal problems.'

Other testosterone products include Tostrelle, a testosterone gel, made by Cellegy who sold the rights to Pro Strakan in 2006 and Androsorb cream, being developed by

Novavax, which is already being used to boost testosterone levels in men (see *chapter eight – testosterone*). BioSante is also developing a testosterone gel called LibiGel. The American-based company Vivus is developing Testosterone MDTS, or Testosterone Metered Dose Transdermal Spray to treat low sexual desire. Vivus is awaiting approval from the FDA to proceed with phase III clinical trials.

ALISTA AND FEMPROX

Vivus is also currently testing a cream called Alista to help women with arousal disorder. The company also makes Muse, the ED product for men.

Alista is a formulation of the drug alprostadil, a synthetic version of a prostaglandin E1 which has similar actions as Viagra: it is a naturally occurring vasodilating agent. Vasodilators increase the diameter of blood vessels allowing them to accommodate larger volumes of blood. In other words, the drug may get blood flowing to the genitalia to induce the warm pre-sexual feelings. The drug will be aimed at women who may be interested in sex but feel they are unable to get properly aroused. This can be even more of a problem after a hysterectomy or the menopause.

Vivus unveiled results of a study involving 80 women at an American Urological Association meeting in June 2002 which showed that alprostadil can have an effect on sexual arousal, sensation and lubrication.

NexMed of the US are looking at Femprox, a vasodilator in cream form. The company announced results of a 372-patient study in China at the congress for the European Society for Sexual Medicine in December 2005. Patients reported increased arousal success rate of up to 41.9 per cent.

FOOTNOTE:

Although Viagra may not be the answer to FSD, there is a possibility that the drug may have a spin-off effect and help women with fertility problems to have children. Studies suggest that it may improve blood flow to the uterus, increasing the thickness of the womb lining.

The research has been conducted at the Sher Institute for Reproductive Medicine in Nevada, USA.

In the study, 73 infertile women, who were undergoing IVF treatment, were given specially designed Viagra suppositories for between three and ten days. The drug therapy was stopped about two days before eggs were harvested for fertilisation and implantation into the uterus. Successful implantation of an embryo was much more likely in the women using Viagra – almost one in three of them had successful implantation, compared to just two per cent of a non-Viagra group, according to the medical journal *Fertility and Sterility*.

Viagra probably helps dilate blood vessels and seems to promote growth of the lining of the uterus without side-effects.

Doctors caution that women who are having problems getting pregnant should not experiment with the drug unsupervised. And women involved in UK trials of Viagra have been told they should not be planning to conceive if they take the drug at this stage.

SCENTUELLE
CST Medical — who also make the Vielle clitoral stimulator — launched Scentuelle patches in 2005. The patch is designed to be worn on the wrist and contains a combination of aromas that create smell molecules that mimic the size, shape and electrical charge of dopamine molecules.

In trials, half of subjects with hypoactive sexual desire disorder reported that sniffing the patch regularly boosted their sex drive, according to findings presented to the International Society for the Study of Women's Sexual Health in 2006.

At the time of writing Scentuelle was not yet available to buy in stores. It can be purchased online at **www.vielle.info/scentuelle** or by calling 0871 911 1746 and costs from £19.95 for 30 patches, plus postage and packaging.

ZESTRA
Zestra arousal oil is a blend of borage seed oil, evening primrose oil, angelica extract, coleus extract and vitamins C and E for application to the genitalia.

Zestra Laboratories Inc. claim that the oil is the only product available that can be used to treat a broad range of sexual problems. Results of a trial published in the *Journal of Sex and Marriage Therapy* in 2003 showed that Zestra increased sexual sensation, arousal, pleasure and satisfaction in women with and without sexual arousal difficulties. Subjects included women suffering sexual side-effects from menopause and medications such as antidepressants and oral contraceptives. However, this manufacturer-funded research included just 20 women.

Zestra costs £14.99 for six sachets and is available to order from **www.zestraforwomen.co.uk** or by calling 0845 658 8877.

Nasal sprays
APORMORPHINE
Apormorphine may help improve both desire and arousal problems in women in order to give a 'sexual buzz' or high. This is a drug well-known to medicine and is used to treat Parkinson's disease. It has also been shown to increase erectile response in men and assists with increased desire by changing dopamine levels in the brain.

Oliver Gillie in his book *Regaining Potency* (Self-Help Direct, 1997) predicted that in the future it will probably be used together with drugs like Viagra — with one drug working on the brain and the other on the blood flow to the penis in men or the clitoris in women. Pharmacia, bought by Pfizer in 2003, is working on a nasal spray version. Meanwhile interesting new trials are going on in the UK.

Ian Russell is a urology nurse in Scotland whose interest began with male libido problems. Eight years ago he developed an interest in FSD.

He knew apormorphine had an effect in males with ED. He said: 'It was tested with men and found that 60% responded, recording a sexual buzz and its ability to affect desire. We wondered what the impact would be for women.' He said that unlike drugs such as Viagra, apormorphine, however, appears to act on the brain, on the para-ventricular cerebral cortex.'

Russell has run a small trial involving just 10 women with no placebos, over 18 weeks. Initially patients were given two tablets twice a week. 'The first time the doses were too small, then they were adjusted, and we started to get a response from women who were reporting a 'sexual high'. When we moved up a notch and they had pills on Monday, Wednesday and Friday they increased their response and their interest in sexual activity. Apormorphine not only acts on the brain but stimulates vaginal congestion. It is a very simple and quite an old drug,' he said. Russell arranged another trial during 2003, involving 100 patients in Scotland. This trial was placebo controlled and the results showed that apormorphine did have a positive effect on female libido. Research is ongoing and Russell is also conducting clinical trials of testosterone gels. No studies have been done on the impact of apormorphine on fertility.

PT 141 – ANOTHER POTENTIAL 'DESIRE' DRUG.

The name refers to the project number given to the potential treatment being developed by Palatin Technologies, a biopharmaceutical company, and King Pharmaceuticals Inc, in conjunction with researchers from Concordia University in Montreal, Canada.

It is a synthetic hormone said to spark desire and is thought to work directly on the central nervous system, making the brain send messages to the nerves in the sexual organs. It may work to boost blood flow to the clitoris making sexual intercourse and orgasm easier. The first trials were conducted on women at the Centre for Studies in Behavioural Neurobiology within the department of psychology at Concordia University. Professor Jim Pfaus, a senior researcher, said: 'These studies examined whether PT-141 would facilitate sexual arousal in women watching a 'female-centric' erotic videoclip, and were conducted in a double-blind trial.

'The drug produced a marked facilitation of vaginal blood volume while women viewed the clip. I also know that some of these women volunteered that they felt aroused and horny while under the influence of the drug, although sexual desire was not examined specifically in this set of studies (and who knows whether they would have felt that way anyway after watching the clip).

An earlier study found that female rats given PT-141 'actively solicited sexual contact from the males'. It also increased the female rats' desire to mate. Dr Annette Shadiack, director of the company's biological research programme, said the results showed that the product 'has a potential to offer a unique treatment'.

PT-141 is a peptide analogue of the neuropeptides hormone called a-melanocyte stimulating hormone (a-MSH). The receptors for these molecules (called melanocortin receptors) play a role in several natural behaviours – notably appetite and sexual arousal. Recent research suggests that if the melanocortin receptors in the brain are stimulated it has an impact on sexual function.

Vaginal tablets and creams

VAGIFEM
An oestroidal vaginal tablet designed to combat dryness and pain on intercourse, it is available on NHS prescription for women who don't want traditional HRT. It is a tablet the size of a junior aspirin delivered high into the vagina with a pencil-type applicator.

HRT with extras

LIVIAL
It contains tibolone, a synthetically produced hormone that has a mix of oestrogen and testosterone-like substances. It is only prescribed in the menopause, once periods have stopped for a year, and is already used for osteoporosis and HRT. It has also been found to improve mood and libido.

ESTRATEST
This contains both testosterone and oestrogen but is not yet available in Europe. It is widely prescribed in the US and has been found to boost libido in some women.

LASOFOXIFENE
Another type of HRT (a SERM, or selective oestrogen receptor modulator), Lasofoxifene is being investigated for its benefits for FSD in women in their 40s, 50s and 60s in the US and the UK as part of an international research programme. In phase III clinical trials at George Washington University in 2005 women reported fewer symptoms of dyspareunia after taking Lasofoxifene for 12 weeks.

OESTROGEN RINGS
Oestrogen is thought to improve clitoral sensitivity in women. In the US and UK a vaginal ring called Estring delivers low-dose oestrogen which might help women with complaints of vaginal dryness. It is available on an NHS prescription.

HERBS SUPPLEMENTS AND POTIONS
Herbal remedies help some women. Ensure you buy from reputable sources and tell your GP if you are on other medication, as some herbal products can inter-react with traditional medicines. Herbal supplements that that may help include **black cohosh, dong quai, ginseng and red clover**. You will need to try them for at least four weeks before seeing results. There have been some very small-scale trials but as yet there is no conclusive scientific evidence that shows whether they are truly beneficial, or not, for female sexual dysfunction.

VIGOREX FEMME

Contains avena sativa (green oats) and saw palmetto, and claims to increase sexual thoughts, desire and enjoyment, as well as boosting overall energy levels. Whether saw palmetto makes a difference has yet to be shown.

L-ARGANINE

A precursor to nitric oxide, this is an amino acid sold in health food shops and promoted by several internet sites. L-arganine helps relax the smooth muscle but has not been tested in large-scale clinical trials. The claims are that it produces a 'vigorous tingle'.

One supplement that includes the chemical is **Veromax** which also contains extracts of the South East Asian jujube date, ginseng, gingko, and soya isoflavones. It's available from Boots at £32.99 for a one-month supply or via mail order: tel 0208 340 3886.

Vibrance cream, which recently launched in the UK, also contains L-Arginine. It is the first sexual arousal cream developed by gynaecologists. Trials at the University of West Virginia in 2005 found that sexual arousal was increased in all subjects when applied to the clitoris prior to sex and 30% who had previously been unable to climax for a significant period of time experienced orgasm. Vibrance costs £24.99 for 10 applications and is available from Boots and **www.indigohealth.co.uk**.

Other L-argine products are: **Viacrème** (it also includes menthol), and **Dream Cream**, both available over the internet. (Try **www.healthsuperstore.com** or **www.dreamcream.com**).

These are said to be a 'natural topical creams which are applied to the genitals to act as a stimulant to the soft tissues and create a 'cool, tingling' sensation. The manufacturers claim this can result in greater orgasmic pleasure and help induce orgasm for women having difficulty.

SAW PALMETTO

Claimed to be the herbal 'Viagra', this is a palm tree that grows in North America and the West Indies and has long been said to be a male aphrodisiac. The plant may influence both testosterone and oestrogen in the body and relax smooth muscle.

WILD MEXICAN YAM

Thought to mimic the effects of progesterone. Some researchers believe it provides chemicals needed by the body to make DHEA, a hormone made in the adrenal glands which acts as building block for sex hormones.

HERBAL VX

Made by Swiss Health, this contains the Peruvian plant muira puama plus ginseng, both thought to have had some success in improving libido. (**www.elixirhealth.co.uk**)

YOHIMBINE OR AFRICAN TREE BARK

An 'improved' version of this herb made from African tree bark has been found to increase vaginal blood flow in postmenopausal women and may be a treatment option for female sexual arousal disorder, according to researchers from the University of Texas at Austin, working with association with NitroMed, Inc. The product is said to work by dilating the blood vessels in women's genitalia while also improving blood flow into the region. The Texas team conducted a study of NMI-870 and compared it with regular yohimbine and with a placebo.

'We found that the drug was most effective after 60 minutes,' said psychologist Dr Cindy Meston in an interview with Reuters Health.

'The litmus test will be measuring the effects of the medication in an actual sexual situation. Our work was done in the lab. We can show that NMI-870 works on the vaginal responses. Now we would like to determine if it increases a woman's sexual satisfaction.'

To date, NMI-870 has only been tested in postmenopausal women who had difficulty becoming aroused. Meston hopes testing will be expanded to other ages. NitroMed, Inc. has been developing nitric oxide-enhanced medications since 1997. Researchers have developed a similar version of nitric oxide-enhanced yohimbine for men with erectile dysfunction, that is also in clinical trials.

The gadgets

EROS-CTD (CLITORAL THERAPY DEVICE)

This is the first product to be licensed for FSD treatment in America by the US Food and Drug Administration (FDA). It is now available in the UK from Beecourse Ltd (www.eros-therapy.co.uk). It costs £199.75 and it works to increase blood flow by creating a vacuum around the clitoris – the mechanism is similar to that of the male vacuum erection device which causes penile blood flow engorgement.

The device is designed for women who suffer from diminished vaginal lubrication, low clitoral sensation, poor sexual satisfaction, and a reduced ability to experience orgasm. The device consists of a battery operated vacuum and a disposable cup which draws blood into the clitoris. A clinical test showed that of 15 women who experienced arousal problems, all experienced an improved sensation, seven had more orgasms, 12 more satisfaction, and 11 more lubrication.

VIELLE

This is a product launched in the UK and Europe in 2003 by CST Medical, a company set up in 1999 to make products for women with FSD conditions. Vielle costs £7.49 for a pack of three and is available over the counter at Boots, Superdrug and Tesco.

The PVC-made device is a clitoral stimulator that fits over a (male or female) finger, and has nodules on the end. The product has undergone trials set up by sexual medicine expert Prof. Alan Riley. As a result, the company claims Vielle makes orgasms more intense, and much quicker and easier to reach. It may help women who have had long-term orgasm problems such as those who find it hard to attain orgasm and then 'give up' because of the time it takes. CST can be contacted on 01274 587400. **www.vielle.info**

EMOTIONAL BLISS (EB)
Run by psychosexual counsellor Julia Cole, this company supplies new age, modern vibrators designed by women for women. They look unlike the traditional vibrators and are designed to sit over the clitoris. **www.emotionalbliss.com**

FPSALES.COM
This internet site is run by a branch of the Family Planning Association (known as the fpa) and offers a Sexware range of vibrators and sex aids in a 'non-sensational' way. The company says that all products featured on their website have been examined by a medical practitioner with nearly 30 years' experience in sexual health matters.

The SexWare range has the support of Relate, Spinal Injuries Association, British Association for Sexual and Relationship Therapy and Age Concern. Their medical advisor says: 'Sexuality is an integral part of every person, male and female of all ages. Expression of sexuality is a very personal matter and for an individual to have choice of expression is very important.

'We hope this range will be helpful in this context. For some it will be a means of adding to sexual pleasure and expression, others may find it helpful in enabling them to express their sexuality where there may be some physical sexual difficulty. We hope it will be valuable in helping you to express your sexuality as an individual, or as a couple.' tel: **0870 444 5116**; website: **www.fpsales.com**

VAGINAL TRAINERS
Designed to improve strength of pelvic floor muscles, these are available from some pharmacies or try **www.pelvictoner.co.uk** – they cost around £30.

Surgery
VAGINAL REJUVENATION
In an interview with the New York Times in November 2004, Dr. V. Leroy Young, chairman of the emerging trends task force for the American Society of Plastic Surgeons, spoke of the rapidly growing demand for surgical procedures to improve the look of the genitals and enhance sexual satisfaction.

The most popular are tightening of the vaginal muscles, or vaginoplasty, and reduction of the labia minora, called labiaplasty. In the past such procedures were reserved for problems like incontinence, congenital malformations or injuries related to childbirth. Now they are being promoted by some plastic surgeons as 'vaginal rejuvenation' for ordinary women.

Although most surgeons offering the procedure in the US stress that vaginal rejuvenation is not a treatment for sexual dysfunction, it is widely marketed as a way of increasing sexual pleasure. Anecdotal evidence suggests that a small but increasing number of women are seeking vaginal rejuvenation to correct sexual problems caused by the weakening of vaginal muscles after childbirth.

Until recently women in the UK seeking genital surgery had to go abroad. In October 2006, the UK Laser Vaginal Rejuvenation Centre opened in Harley Street, London. The centre is the first clinic of its kind in the UK. At the time of writing 16 patients had undergone treatment at the Centre and more than 50 had attended consultation.

Laser Vaginal Rejuvenation is said to enhance vaginal muscle tone, strength, and control, decrease the internal and external vaginal diameters and build up and strengthen the perineal body. However, gynaecologists warn that intercourse can be painful if the vaginal muscles over corrected and other possible risks include painful scarring or nerve damage that could result in loss of sensation.

The cost of vaginal rejuvenation starts at around £2800.

Stuck for words?
WHAT TO SAY TO THE DOCTOR
It can be embarrassing bringing up the subject of sex at a consultation with a doctor. But the advice of health professionals is to be as frank and open as possible.

- 'Don't go to your doctor with a complaint about a sprained ankle and then say at the end, well, really I have a sexual problem,' advises Dr David Goldmeier, who runs a sexual health clinic at St Mary's Hospital, Paddington.
- Be frank – say that you are distressed about a sexual problem. Write down how you feel in note form before the consultation. Take some literature – maybe this book – with you and say 'this is how I feel'.
- Avoid using technical terms or jargon. Stick to plain language about how you feel and the impact it is having on you and your relationship.
- If you previously had a happy sex life and now find you cannot enjoy orgasm tell your doctor about the change, and say that you want help.
- If your doctor remains unsympathetic contact the Impotence Association and ask for the name of a sympathetic doctor in your area.
- Don't forget Relate, they have sexual therapists in most regions of the country and the therapist may know of a good doctor in your area.
- You may even find an understanding doctor at the local GU clinic (genito-urinary).
- Not all gynaecologists will be interested in a sexual problem.
- Therapists will want to know the root cause of the problem – if it is linked to an experience that has then led to changed behaviour.
- Become acquainted with your anatomy.

What the Sexual Dysfunction Association says:

Mary Davern, of the Sexual Dysfunction Association, said their helpline receives calls from women who say they are experiencing difficulty with their sex life. The calls come from women who are very distressed. Some have lost interest in sex, others experience pain during sex and some are unable to have sex. Often, as a result of this their relationship is under a great deal of strain.

The association advises women that their first port of call should be their GP. Many have already spoken to their doctor but in a lot of cases they were unable to help.

One way of helping yourself, she advises, is to take some information about FSD along to the doctor and show it to them, saying 'This is how I feel, this is the pain I am feeling, this is what I am trying to explain to you.' Often women cannot say the words, said Mary – especially if they receive an unsympathetic approach the first time around.

The SDA has a list of sympathetic doctors, so if your GP proves unhelpful, they should be able to supply the name of a clinic or GP in your area who has expressed an interest in FSD and its investigation. Already more GPs and specialists – in different branches of medicine such as urology and gynaecology – are available to help women. There has been some eradication of the embarrassment, which has prevented these conversations and consultations from taking place in the past.

Where do I find treatment?

Doctors in a variety of fields are becoming more interested in FSD. This is helped by the fact there are now international conferences on the subject, and an influx of cash available for research flowing from drug companies.

The drug companies have a major interest in developing awareness of FSD – the market place is potentially massive, worth billions. If they can develop a drug that really helps they will strike gold. FSD specialists are emerging in two distinct branches of health care: gynaecology and genito-urinary medicine. But it will depend on the interest of the specialists in your particular area and unfortunately there are still no guarantees your problem will be taken seriously.

If your problem is caused by some type of vulval pain then make contact with the Vulval Pain Society (see *chapter six – painful sex*). It is expected that the first FSD medicines will become available in the next five years for selected groups of affected women which should mean that family doctors will be encouraged to find out more about FSD and get to know what drugs are available.

There are already moves afoot to have 'sexual medicine' recognised by its own faculty or fellowship – all this debate will help to spread the word amongst health professionals that FSD conditions really do exist and trouble women. In the meantime, expect a rise of 'alternative' products such as herbs and supplements as interest in the subject of FSD grows. Finally, I like this comment from the Australian Women's Forum published in April 2001 in its summary of available treatments. *Caring, nurturing, supportive partner who knows where the clitoris is. Cost: Priceless. Not available on prescription.*

Reference

[1]Kaplan, S. A., *et al.* Safety and efficacy of sildenafil on postmenopausal women with sexual dysfunction. *Urology* 1999. **53** (3): 481-6.

[2]Diamond, L.E., et al. An Effect on the Subjective Sexual Response in Premenopausal Women with Sexual Arousal Disorder by Bremelanotide (PT-141), a Melanocortin Receptor Agonist. *Journal of Sexual Medicine* 2006. (3):628–638.

8

testosterone – the hormone of desire?

CAUSES OF TESTOSTERONE DEFICIENCY

■ A decline with age
■ Following an operation to remove the ovaries as part of a hysterectomy levels fall by as much as 50%.
■ Some treatments for endometriosis may affect testosterone levels.
■ Chemotherapy and radiotherapy may also have an impact.
■ The contraceptive pill
■ An Australian doctor found that giving women intra muscular testosterone after a hysterectomy or 'surgical menopause' helped women feel more composed, elated and energetic.

Testosterone is an androgen, the male sex hormone that is also secreted in smaller amounts by the ovaries and adrenal glands in women. It has been nicknamed the fuel of love and the hormone of desire because of its positive influence on the sex drive. It is now recognised that it can also affect mood, well-being, energy and vitality in some women.

As women age, their levels of testosterone fall considerably. There is a growing body of scientific literature focusing on the role of androgens in maintaining women's health and well-being and increasing recognition of a disorder known as FADS – Female Androgen Deficiency Syndrome.

There are now plenty of women who maintain they have had their love lives restored through testosterone implants which gradually secrete the hormone, over several months, into the bloodstream. One woman has been treated by a London menopause clinic for 15 years, returning every six months for a new pellet to be implanted.

At present the only licensed testosterone product for women is this implant, which is inserted into thighs or buttocks or the lower part of the anterior abdominal wall. But Procter and Gamble's testosterone patch was set to be launched at the time of writing.

In the meantime, some women have been crossing the Channel on 'love trips' to pick up supplies of a testosterone gel produced in France called Andractim which is available if a prescription is given by a UK doctor. The product is not licensed in the UK but is available through French and Swiss pharmacies.

Malcolm Whitehead who runs the menopause clinic at King's College Hospital said women are going over for lunch in France on day trips and picking up their prescription on the way home.

The gel is also licensed in Switzerland. Women prefer using a gel because it's easier to apply – once a day – and there is none of the potential soreness and bruising associated with having the 'desire' hormone implant.

In the UK, the licensed implant 'drip feeds' testosterone into the body for up to a year, although six-eight months is more usual. At the start of treatment, when the implant is first inserted, levels of testosterone in the body can climb to above the normal female range and brings the risk of side effects – increased facial hair, a rise in lipid levels in the blood which could increase risks of heart disease, acne and greasy skin.

There is a hope that soon androgen therapy will become far more accessible through GPs or family planning clinics – at present only a handful of clinics in the country offer the testosterone implant therapy.

You could in the future have the case of a woman with an oestrogen patch on one buttock and an androgen patch on the other, said Mr Whitehead.

The problem at the moment is that few gynaecologists are aware of the androgen story in relation to women's sexual disinterest – and there is at present no easy way for GPs to determine testosterone levels in women.

Testosterone is only likely to help a certain number of women – but for those who find it helps, it is life-enhancing.

All plasma tests would have to be done by a hospital pathology lab – and it is an expensive process. Malcolm Whitehead's clinic inserts about 20 testosterone implants a week. Women, he says, come back when their implant runs out asking for more because their libido has once again diminished.

Androgen deficiency was originally identified in women who had undergone hysterectomy and removal of the ovaries. But it has been subsequently found that a low dose of testosterone can help improve an ailing sexual drive in both pre- and post-menopausal women, and also treat other conditions such as pre-menstrual tension and importantly, the all-consuming listlessness and fatigue experienced by so many women.

The Jean Hailes Foundation in Australia is one of the centres leading this work. Dr Susan Davis, the research director who has been treating women with severe loss of sexual feelings with 50mg testosterone implants, says she has been getting some 'unbelievable results'. She is regularly sent 'large numbers' of women by GPs and other specialists. Most of the women, she says, have had their ovaries removed but there are others who develop arousal problems after starting on HRT. She says this is because HRT can further lower biologically-available testosterone.

Women with testosterone deficiency will complain about not being bothered by sex, or say: 'I can't bear anyone to touch me.' But the message is more one of a loss of interest rather than a dysfunction – and some experts now believe that low testosterone levels should be classified as a mood disorder rather than a sexual dysfunction. Women treated with testosterone often report improved sexual motivation, desire fantasy and arousal, as well as satisfaction and orgasm.

But testosterone treatment for women is still considered controversial by some doctors. There may be risks and unwanted side effects unless the dosage is very carefully managed. Dr Davis says that no woman will die of androgen deficiency but links between its depletion and depression and feelings of well-being have been established.

There are few controlled studies which show a clear benefit – although there is

---

CASE HISTORY

Until the age of 32, Kate says she never felt any need for a sexual outlet, never experienced sexual daydreams and never recognised sexual arousal. She had a life-long absence of a sex drive.

With two different boyfriends, she found sex was painful, uncomfortable and she only went through the motions because she wanted the companionship rather than to satisfy any sexual need. The first time Kate went to bed with a boyfriend was a disaster: it was simply too painful to consummate the relationship. It took a few drinks before Kate and her boyfriend felt relaxed enough to try again, and they had to use lubrication jelly. A second relationship five years later was again unsuccessful. It lasted just nine months and although Kate participated in sex (again with the help of extra lubrication) she says she never felt sexually excited. At 28, Kate went to a sex therapist and was given a series of 'self-pleasuring exercises' to complete. She felt no erotic sensations at all and thought it all a waste of time. After nine months she stopped seeing her therapist as it was simply not helping. At 32, Kate was referred to the sexual dysfunction clinic at St. George's Hospital in London where an examination revealed that she had a very small clitoris, and labia minor. Tests showed oestrogen and thyroid levels were normal but a further blood test revealed a clue – her testosterone levels were on the low side but more interestingly she also had a very low level of DHT (dihydrotestosterone), an active component of testosterone. It has long been recognised that androgens (the sex hormones which include testosterone) play a major part in the sex drive. This finding pinpointed a precise abnormality. Kate was prescribed a DHT gel which was obtained by her doctor from France where it is used to treat breast enlargement in men. After just eight weeks of treatment Kate experienced for the first time a tingling in her clitoris which had also increased slightly in size. Using self-pleasuring techniques she had been taught earlier, Kate experienced orgasm for the first time. At the age of 35, she now has a boyfriend and is enjoying a normal sexual relationship with him. Kate was one of 19 women who with a complete absence of sex drive who were being studied by Prof. Alan Riley. Levels of seven different hormones in these women were analysed in detail. Kate was the only one to show low level of DHT. Her case is considered very unusual. Prof. Riley said: 'This case is very important because it shows for the first time that a loss of sex drive has a physical cause. This woman showed a quite dramatic improvement after treatment. However, because only one of the 19 women studied has shown this abnormal level of DHT the assumption is that it is a cause, but perhaps not a common cause of the problem.'

plenty of positive clinical feedback. But Dr Davis says the dose is all important: she rarely gives more than 50mg implants. Higher doses could lead to problems. She also closely monitors the woman's levels, which provide information for individual management. Dr Davis says: 'I have never seen virilisation in a woman I have treated and I have been giving testosterone for more than 15 years.'

In the normal course of events, women's androgen levels fall as they age. They do not fall dramatically at the menopause (as oestrogen levels do) but there is a gradual decline. The availability of androgen in the body is also thought to be influenced by sex hormone-binding globulins – and both ageing and the use of the contraceptive pill increase plasma levels of SHBG, reducing the amounts of testosterone available to target tissues.

Dr Davis has concluded that many older women who complain of a lack of sexual drive are in fact suffering from androgen deficiency. In one of her defining studies organised over two years, Dr Davis studied the effects of oestrogen implants upon sexuality. Some implants contained oestrogen alone, while others contained a combination of oestrogen and testosterone. The group treated with oestrogen and testosterone experienced a greater improvement in sexuality compared to the oestrogen-only group. Dr Davis found that this combination also improved libido.

The results of the work, she says, establishes testosterone as having a 'genuine and persistent treatment effect' and she is currently trying to analyse the proportion of women with sexual arousal and desire difficulties who might benefit.

In a report[1] submitted to the *Journal of Impotence Research*, Dr Davis writes: 'In conclusion, this study reaffirms that added testosterone enhances sexuality in post-menopausal women and can be of significant benefit for women experiencing low libido despite adequate oestrogen replacement.' Testosterone treatment, says Dr Davis, should be considered for all symptomatic post-menopausal women especially those who have experienced an early menopause.

However the long-term effects of testosterone therapy upon vascular function has not been deeply studied in normal healthy women. Dr Davis is now looking at blood vessel function in post-menopausal women who are receiving testosterone replacement implants as part of their normal hormone replacement regimen.

Meanwhile, researchers at Yale University in the US have also found that HRT with added testosterone leads to an improvement in sexual functioning – with notable improvements in sexual desire, fantasy and response and a decrease of painful sex compared with oestrogen-only hormonal treatment.

They also found that vaginal blood flow increased (which physiologically helps with lubrication problems) compared with the oestrogen-only group. In conclusion, the researchers suggest that women who have been on HRT for a year or so (particularly after a hysterectomy) may benefit from ART to help restore feelings of sexual desire.

In a question and answer session at an international conference on impotence problems in Cape Cod, Dr Davis told a discussion panel that there is a pattern among women who complain of sexual dysfunction and who have an androgen deficiency.

'There is a constant repetitive pattern in what these women say. A classic case is a woman who was 35 and had had endometriosis and both ovaries removed. She is on increasing doses of oestrogen but still says 'I feel lousy, I felt flat, I'm tired, I have no sexual desire.' Every woman says the same thing. The non-responders (those who do not respond to ART) do not come out with the same story.'

Dr Davis also highlights other groups of affected women. 'I have seen a number of young girls who have had chemotherapy for adolescent leukaemia and women who have had a range of different chemotherapies who say they are sick and tired of being told they are depressed, and that they are tired because of their chemotherapy or because their kids are getting them down or because their marriage might be on the rocks: in fact they have a discrete androgen deficiency. We all have lifestyle stress and pressure but often you can help these women greatly by simply giving them a little bit of androgen.'

Are you androgen deficient?
The common symptoms are:
- excessive tiredness – more than you might expect from other contributing factors
- feelings of listlessness
- low sex drive or desire difficulties
- loss of pubic hair
- loss of muscle mass

You are more at risk:
- if you have had your ovaries removed and are being treated with oestrogen – but with no improvement in well-being or libido
- are on the pill
- are menopausal

Further information:
Susan Davis MBBS, FRACP PhD, Director of Research, The Jean Hailes Foundation, Victoria, Australia (www.jeanhailes.org.au).

Menopause Clinic and Gynae-Endocrine service, King's College Hospital, Denmark Hill, London (call 0203 299 2785 or visit www.kch.nhs.uk).

References
[1]Davis. S. R. The role of androgens and the menopause in the female sexual response. International Journal of Impotence Research 1998. **10**: 82-83.
See also: Davis. S. R. the Clinical use of Androgens in Female sexual Disorders. Journal of Sexual and Marital Therapy 1998. **24** (3): 153-63.

9

looking after yourself

Improving your health

It seems only commonsense that sex lives can benefit from general healthy living guidelines. But it is now official: research in the States has found that women with low sexual desire can benefit from exercise – or, indeed, anything which stimulates the sympathetic nervous system, causing an increase in heart rate and blood pressure. Twenty minutes of vigorous exercise can improve the blood flow to the genital region and therefore lubrication – with the most marked effect 15 to 30 minutes after you have finished exercising.

Rather than take a bubble bath to relax the advice now is to get out to the gym and rev up your body and do something 'arousing' like pounding the treadmill. You will feeling better about yourself in general.

Looking after your body makes you feel better about yourself. And when you reconnect with your body you can start to reconnect with needs and desires, the pleasures and pain of life. And this can help you to feel sexual again.

Exercise

Less than half of all women over the age of 19 exercise regularly, according to medical researchers. This is despite the fact that exercise can promote an overall sense of well-being, counter stress, reduce the side-effects of the menopause and the risk of the bone crippling disease, osteoporosis. Research has shown that exercise enhances the physiological sexual response, causing a greater flow of blood to the genitals – a vital requirement in the physical arousal process and lubrication of the vagina.

Dr Cindy Meston, a psychologist at the University of Texas, has conducted studies[1] investigating the effect of stimulating the sympathetic nervous system through exercise before exposure to erotic stimuli. She found that the sexually-driven engorgement of the genitals and blood flow to the vagina is heightened 15 to 30 minutes after exercise – and that this happens in sexually functioning women just as well as it does in those who report low sexual desire problems.

However, there is a quite different result in women who complain of anorgasmia, the failure to attain orgasm. In studies these women show no equivalent increase of blood flow to the genitals after exercise and exposure to erotic stimulation.

Dr Meston's studies suggest for the first time that there is a physiological component to anorgasmia. She says: 'Until now it has been assumed that anorgasmia is the result of a number of psychological issues, e.g. religious concerns, fear of losing control, anxiety, relationship issues, a lack of sufficient stimuli or sexual inexperience - that is, not knowing how to have an orgasm. My study suggests that, in addition, there may be a purely physical element.'

The problems could be related to the functioning of the nervous system of the supply of blood to the genitals and vagina.

Important conclusions from this work

- exercise may help your body prepare for sex – especially if you plan to have sex 15 to 30 minutes afterwards
- exercise may particularly help women with sexual desire problems. Stimulation of the sympathetic nervous system, which causes your blood pressure to rise, the heart to beat faster and digestive processes to slow down, can influence the physiological sexual response in women with sexual desire problems.
- anything that stimulates the sympathetic nervous system may help. Dr Meston suggests other things, apart from exercise, could include going to see a scary or action movie, watching a comedy, enjoying a roller coaster ride – perhaps even drinking a shot of espresso.

Dr Meston noted the improved physiological response after exercise in three sets of trials involving 90 women – but she also found that the women with a heightened response to sexual stimulation after exercise were not aware of what was happening. This failure to recognise what is happening in the genitals (the feelings associated with blood flow to the vagina and clitoris) and linking it with sexual arousal is a common story among sexologists. It poses the question – could women be helped to identify their sexual responses by monitoring them through a small biofeedback machine which would reveal the increased blood flow? At present no such instrument exists for home use.

Dr Meston says affected women would benefit from being taught to associate increases in their sympathetic nervous system with a sexually pleasurable experience by providing them with feedback on their genital responses which shows when the sympathetic nervous system is activated they have a greater sexual response.

Women could then be taught to associate these signals of increases in heart rate and blood pressure with positive thoughts of becoming 'more sexual' as opposed to negative anxiety-related performance thoughts. This might involve teaching women to associate increases in the sympathetic nervous system with a sexually pleasurable experience.

Apart from these findings, which may lead to new treatments for women with low sexual desire, exercise will enhance your overall sense of well-being. When you exercise the body releases endorphins, natural opiate-like substances, into the bloodstream which create a sense of mild euphoria. You will sleep better and feel more relaxed generally, and this may help you to feel less tense about sex.

Be creative when it comes to exercise: there are plenty of different dance classes to try. A combination of swimming, the gym, an aerobics class and walking will not only help you stay fit but can be fun too. Making time, however, is often difficult. Consider sharing the costs of a personal trainer with a friend or two and start the day early with a workout session. Most swimming pools or health clubs open early for pre-work swims.

Research suggests that post-menopausal women particularly benefit from exercise – it has been shown to improve mood and decrease stress levels. Stress exacerbates menopausal symptoms so anything you can do to alleviate stress levels may help with hot flushes and possibly even a dry vagina, especially if you use some of the other self-help ideas found elsewhere in this book in conjunction with an exercise plan.

In trials, pain in intercourse was helped in a group of women who took HRT and exercise rather than just exercise alone. However, if you don't want to take HRT, or you are unable to for health reasons, exercise combined with a good eating plan may help to alleviate other problems, and should certainly encourage you to feel better about yourself and boost your self-esteem. You may then be encouraged to take the next step and address your sexual problems.

There are plenty of other good reasons for exercise: being active benefits the heart by increasing the way oxygen is delivered and used and also helps to keep weight at a reasonable level. An increase in exercise will result in an increase in the number of calories burnt up by the body – the key to an exercise plan is to carry it through consistently. Twice a week every week is far better than five times a week for a month and then nothing for a month.

Other health problems

After menopause, women's risk of arterial disease rises as they lose the protective oestrogen factors. A diet high in fat will contribute to arterial disease and the formation of atheroma. In men this can affect arteries which feed the penis and affect erections. Early research suggests that women can also suffer from arterial damage affecting the genital region.

SMOKING

There is enormous pressure upon people to stop smoking – and although it sounds like a cracked record, giving up really can improve your health. Smoking has a terrible effect upon blood vessels and will contribute to a narrowing of the arteries.

OVERWEIGHT

Being overweight can affect not only your self-esteem and your feelings of sexuality but you are also more likely to suffer from blood vessel disease and be at greater risk of heart disease. Losing weight can improve cholesterol levels in affected women and can help to control high blood pressure. But losing weight takes commitment, determination and motivation. Rather than dieting religiously you may benefit from reducing your 'fear of food' by eating well, three times a day and concentrating on a good balance of fruit, vegetable, lean protein and complex carbohydrates, and eating less sugary and high fat foods. A woman's relationship with food is often associated with emotional peaks and troughs and you may find that there is also a link between food and sex: if you are in control of your diet rather than food having control over you, you may feel better about yourself as a sexual partner. Keeping everything in balance – food, stress levels and the right amount of exercise – can mean lifestyle changes. Even when these are in place don't expect perfection: we all lapse from grace from time to time because it is human nature to want to indulge ourselves.

ALCOHOL

Excessive alcohol can damage nerves in many parts of the body – in men it has been shown to affect nerves to the penis, so there is every reason to assume that women can also lose genital sensation as a result of too much alcoholic drink.

But drinking in moderation may often improve our mood for sex: there is something about a glass of champagne before bed on a special occasion. Drinking in moderation may temporarily alleviate feelings of tension or anxiety – although it can never be the solution to any sexual problem. If you find that you need to drink before sex then you will have to examine why you feel like this, and then consider ways to address the problem.

References

[1]Meston, C. M., Gorzalka, B. B. The effects of sympathetic activation on physiological and subjective sexual arousal in women. *Behaviour Research and Therapy* 1995. **33** (6): 651-664.
Meston, C. M., Gorzalka, B. B. The effects of immediate, delayed and residual sympathetic activation on sexual arousal in women. *Behaviour Research and Therapy* 1996. **34** (2): 143-148.

10

the happiness factor

'The great majority of the reason our marriage split up was because our sex life was so unsatisfactory to him,'
Janine, aged 27.

Improving your sense of worth and self-esteem

Happiness is a vital key to an improved sex life. Happiness with self, partner, home and work life. The fact that so many women have sexual desire problems indicates that in our modern society there is also a high level of unhappiness. Our sexuality and our happiness are often intertwined, influencing the other parts of our lives.

Can we improve the sexual happiness in our lives? Most of us need some help to balance all the strands of our lives and all the constant juggling we have to face. In doing so, we often forget to take time out for ourselves. But if we neglect our well-being, then other areas of our life will be damaged. In this chapter, we list some ideas, which might help to boost the happiness quota. Combined with other approaches mentioned elsewhere, they will help you create the foundation for a happier, more fulfilled sex life.

They are:
- diet for sexual health
- food supplements and aphrodisiacs to improve libido
- exercise techniques to strengthen the pelvic floor and vaginal muscles
- stress relief and relaxation techniques
- finding out what turns you on
- different lovemaking techniques
- releasing inhibitions for a more adventurous love life and learning to 'let go'

Diet: food for love

The western diet, high in fat and sugar, has been found to lower levels of sex hormone-binding globulin which controls how much oestrogen and testosterone is carried around the body. Good, wholesome and ordinary food – not five-minute wonder diets which make outrageous claims – should be the key to healing your sexual problem. If our bodies become frail due to bad health, sex invariably suffers (although poor health does not always have to mean poor sex). A good wholesome diet will help lay the foundations of good health.

Eating foods like grains, milk, eggs, lean meat, chicken, nuts, dried fruit, fish, green vegetables and fish will help boost sex hormone function. Adding foods containing beneficial fatty acids such as those found in mackerel, olive oil and evening primrose oil will also help to improve sex hormone function.

But don't forget the basics: at least five portions of fruit and vegetables a day will provide a cornerstone for health and, for older women, will provide much of the fibre to help keep arteries clear and in good condition.

Calcium-rich foods such as greens and figs should be included in the diets of women from the 20s and 30s age groups to help boost supplies of calcium and help to ward off osteoporosis which will affect one in three women over 50.

Some women experience sugar cravings and are literally 'addicted' to sugar-filled foods. Find out if you have this problem, talk it over with a nutritionist. It may be hard to wean yourself off reaching for cakes and biscuits but a starting point is replacing the high sugar, high fat foods with low fat oat bars, or a slice of rye bread and honey. Keep a high sugar, high fat treat until after a wholesome meal. For advice on beating sugar cravings contact the Natural Health Advisory Service incorporating the Women's Nutritional Advisory Service on 01273 487366. Visit **www.naturalhealthas.com** or write to PO Box 268, Lewes, East Sussex, BN7 1QN.

Bread is a brilliant carbohydrate providing a slow release of energy – there are some wonderful grainy varieties available. Try bread made from rye, oats, corn and rice to ring the changes from wheat-based products. Try making your own – bread makers are much cheaper now than when they originally came onto the market, and there are lovely organic flours available in most large supermarkets. Use honey instead of sugar to make the yeast work, and add olive oil instead of butter for deeply nutritious, easily home-made bread.

Keep coffee and tea to a minimum. Instead opt for camomile or other herbal teas – peppermint is refreshing and fenugreek has a lovely strong flavour, and is also helpful for good digestion. Eat three good meals a day and snack on dried fruit, seeds and nuts but beware of the calorie load.

Cut down on salt which can be detrimental if you are prone to high blood pressure. Oysters are high in zinc and are a traditional aphrodisiac. Try to limit alcohol if you are attempting to boost the nutrient content of your diet.

Give up animal fats where possible, replacing them with soya oil and olive oil, for cooking. But keep fried or deep-fried foods to a minimum – instead stir fry with a minimum of oil for tasty and nutritious vegetarian dishes.

Much more attention is being paid to the benefits for women of eating foods rich in natural phytoestrogens which may be particularly helpful for women about to go through the menopause. Soya products are one of the richest food sources of isoflavones, naturally occurring oestrogen. Soya also contains compounds which may have anti-cancer properties and play a role in minimising many of the symptoms associated with the menopause – including dry vaginas. Soya may also offer some protection against furring of the arteries, heart attacks and strokes.

For further information about phytoestrogens, contact the **Natural Health Advisory Service**.

Supplements for sex

FOOD SUPPLEMENTS

Ginseng is used in traditional Chinese medicine to enhance stamina and ability to cope with tiredness and stress. It may influence the release of nitric oxide which in men is the triggering factor for the blood flow into the penis. If nitric oxide is proven to have the same action upon the erectile tissue in women, then ginseng will prove to be a beneficial aphrodisiac.

In the meantime it has been shown to boost the immune system, and influence carbohydrate and fat metabolism, and the cardiovascular system. Buy authentic ginseng root for the most beneficial effect. In Chinese medicine, ginseng is seen as a great balancer of the body's needs and is often used to increase the vital energy of the body.

Gingko biloba: there is medical interest in its effectiveness for treating sexual problems caused by taking anti-depressants. A study at the University of California showed that women were more responsive to the 'sexually enhancing' effects of gingko

---

NUTRITIONAL THERAPY

Maryon Stewart of the NHAS claims nutritional therapy helps 90% of women revitalise a flagging libido within four to six months. She believes that a nutritional approach can help, particularly if you notice the problems are worse before a period,. 'The body depends on vitamins and minerals to function properly. When under stress there is a significantly increased demand for essential nutrients. Because we lack education about the foods which contain the important nutrients, those increased demands may not be met.'

The NHAS offers a personal dietary programme after a personal evaluation – obtained either through the post or over the phone. Women are asked to list their food and drink intake for a typical week which is analysed for a fee. The NHAS goes on to create a tailor-made programme. The NHAS has clinics in Sussex and London.

biloba than men. The native plant of the Far East generally had a positive effect upon desire, excitement and orgasm. The US study began when it was noticed that an elderly patient taking gingko biloba for memory loss reported improved erections. The Chinese have been using the plant for thousands of years to treat a number of complaints – it is renowned for its ability to improve circulation.

Wild yam contains phytoestrogens and may help women going through the menopause or those whose sex drive is influenced by low progesterone levels.

L-phenylalanine is an amino acid which is said to promote sexual arousal and may help alleviate depression. The best natural sources are soy, proteins, cheese, almonds, peanuts and sesame seeds but you can find it in 500mg supplement form. It is advised that you take it on an empty stomach and not with protein. People with high blood pressure or who suffer from skin cancer are advised not to take this supplement.

St John's Wort is the number one prescription herb for depression in Germany, but it is also thought to be a useful benefit for boosting libido especially when it is linked to depression or anxiety (see *page 83*).

Black cohosh is a herb which has been studied as an alternative therapy to HRT, and is believed to have a balancing effect upon female sex hormones. It might be helpful if you have gone off sex after having a baby or at the time of the menopause.

Angelica is packed with plant hormones and in the Far East is a well-known tonic for women. It is supposed to be particularly good taken at the menopause as a sexual stimulant.

Damiana is a herb grown in Mexico where it is traditionally used to boost women's libido. Its botanical name is Turnera aphrodisiac.

Optivite and **Gynovite** are available from the WNAS – these are specific nutritional supplements. Optivite helps with PMS while Gynovite is for older women.

L-arginine is available as a food supplement from health shops (see *chapter seven – treatments*).

Vitamins and minerals

Magnesium is required for virtually every chemical process in the body. Stress can deplete magnesium levels – and one of the symptoms of a magnesium deficiency is anxiety. Magnesium is necessary for normal hormonal function in the body – and chronic fatigue is often associated with a deficiency. Good natural sources include chocolate, brewer's yeast, brown rice, soyabeans and wholegrain foods. If you drink lots of tea and coffee it can lead to magnesium deficiency.

Zinc is one of the most important trace minerals and is also required for hormonal function and can influence sexual function: but too much can damage to the immune system. A moderate supplement may help boost sex hormone production. Eggs, oysters and seeds all contain zinc.

Vitamin E helps slow the ageing process and helps the development and maintenance of nerves and muscles. Dr David Weeks, a neuropsychologist in Edinburgh, suggests that Vitamin E is the most important vitamin supplement of them all. Vitamin E supplement is a good all-rounder – especially if you smoke because you will be more at risk of being deficient in this vitamin.

The **B vitamins** are important for sex hormone metabolism and maintaining the sex drive.

Sexual chemistry

It is thought that our natural sex drive is controlled by a whole cascade of different chemical and environmental stimuli. There is interaction between our sex hormones, such as oestrogen and testosterone, and metabolic hormones such as adrenaline and oxytocin, with messages fired via neurotransmitters such as serotonin, dopamine, and noradrenaline.

Pheromones, which are signals secreted by men and women, play a part as does the psychological stimulation (sight of a partner) and the physical stimulation from taste and smell. Then there are cultural influences.

Stress is a major libido killer and may contribute to lowered testosterone levels in women – help the body by avoiding stimulants such as caffeine, sugar, nicotine and alcohol but eat protein rich, unprocessed foods to support the body. Excessive stress can also affect thyroid function and low thyroid function is known to have an impact on sexual desire.

Patrick Holford, the supplements guru, suggests seven supplements for better sex:
- B Vitamins
- zinc
- an antioxidant formula that contains CoQ10
- ginseng
- damiana – the central American herb
- muira pauma – a Brazilian Amazon supplement herb
- maca – a Peruvian herb

TRADITIONAL APHRODISIACS

- angelica was used as a potent aphrodisiac in the 18th century
- clove – suggested dose is one or two drops in honey every day
- fennel – a small amount every day drunk as a tea 'improves sex drive'
- ginger – has been used to 'excite the senses' for centuries
- jasmin – Hindus regard this sweet-smelling flower as an aphrodisiac
- chilli – to stimulate the blood circulation

Pelvic floor exercises

Many women associate these exercises with getting back into shape after childbirth – most post-natal classes advise women to do their 'pelvic floors' to help avoid incontinence.

But these beneficial exercises can help to strengthen vaginal muscles enabling them to grip the penis better and to increase stimulation through intercourse. They were devised some 50 years ago by Dr Arnold Kegel. The pelvic floor consists of several layers of muscles and is a trampoline-like structure of muscle and tissues which supports and holds the organs inside the pelvis.

The main support comes from a pair of muscles which, when contracted, pull the rectum, vagina and urethra forward, towards the pubic bone. The muscles form a figure of eight and loop around the vagina and urethra in the front and the rectum at the back. To improve sexual feeling you want to focus particularly on exercising the front part of the muscle, which pulls the vagina upwards.

We all use our pelvic floor muscles without thinking too much about them but because we can't see them like muscles on our arms or legs, they tend to get forgotten unless we have a problem such as incontinence.

Common symptoms of a weak pelvic floor are:
- you may feel nothing during intercourse
- you may have difficulty retaining a tampon
- you may suffer from involuntary incontinence when you laugh, run or sneeze

One way to identify these muscles is to experiment with them during urination. Stopping the urine mid flow is not something that should be done often, but once or twice will help you to identify the muscles concerned. Another way is to insert one or two fingers into the vagina and contract the muscles – easiest done lying down or standing up in the shower with one foot raised. This also help you become more accustomed and knowledgeable about your body.

Once you have identified the pelvic floor muscles, you can then start using and exercising them. By regularly tightening them for a few seconds and then releasing them you will build up their strength. This may also improve orgasm ability. The exercises can be done anywhere at any time. Use triggers such as answering the phone, going upstairs, standing in the bus queue, or switching on the TV or radio to remind yourself to do them.

Stress relief and relaxation

A lack of interest in sex and the feelings of guilt and responsibility towards a partner – the feelings of letting yourself down, as well as your man – can allow tension and stress to infiltrate your life. Stress from work can spill over and linger at home affecting relationships and sex lives. Stress and anxiety can act like a switch – turning off sexual arousal and desire. Learning to relax for sex can be both pleasurable and good for you. The most positive antidote is relaxation. There are three techniques for relaxation and stress relief which may help you get in the mood for sex:

- massage
- aromatherapy
- breathing exercises

You may equally find that simply having a long soak in the bath, taking time out from family worries and troubles (making time in your diary for a swim or a session in the gym, for example) can be equally beneficial. The key is finding time to wind down, and actively removing yourself for a short period from the source of stress.

Massage

Massage is one of the oldest therapies and between lovers can enhance sexuality. Working on your massage techniques with a partner can do wonders for sexual arousal if it is being affected by stress, worry or anger. Prepare a room with soft lighting, music and fragrant smells from perfumed candles or incense sticks so that you create a tranquil, calm atmosphere. Ensure the room is warm and comfortable with a soft rug or blanket on the bed, mattress or couch. A back massage will reduce tension in the muscles. Try applying pressure on either side of the spine working down from the neck to the pelvis. Press in with thumbs and then release. After a tension-releasing session using massage oils ask your partner to try stimulating your nipples and genitals in the same gentle way.

Aromatherapy

This may be particularly helpful if you are suffering from painful intercourse or vaginismus. Jasmin is said to increase feelings of sensuality and ylang ylang to boost libido. They can be used in a massage but you can also infuse a room with their scent by using an aromatherapy vapouriser, or you could add a few drops to a bath as part of your preparation for sex.

Other beneficial oils are bergamot, angelica and lavender. Some oils are believed to stimulate the release of pheromones and stimulate areas in the brain which promote the ability to let go — so aromatherapy may be useful if you are having difficulty achieving

---

HOW TO EXERCISE THE PELVIC FLOOR

Imagine you are riding up in a lift – and as you reach a different level, you tighten and draw up your pelvic floor muscles a little more without losing any of the tension you have already achieved. Then gradually come down again, controlling the muscles as you do.

Try doing 50 a day. Alternatively, lie down on your back or side with legs apart and chest relaxed. Draw up the pelvic floor – you should feel the vagina tighten. Place your hand on the pubic bone and try to tighten the vagina as high as the level of your hand. Hold for a few seconds and relax.

---

orgasm. Relish the sensuous atmosphere that aromatherapy can bring to a room.

Breathing exercises
Learning how to manage your breathing will aid relaxation – correct abdominal breathing can be practiced daily in sessions of 10 or 15 minutes and after a while you will notice an improvement in your well-being. It may help to relax your body before sex or a gentle hugging session, especially if you think about being warm and comfortable at the same time. Put both hands on the tummy and breathe in slowly through the nose, then let as much air out as possible. Do this several times but ensure that when you breathe, it is your abdomen and not your chest which is moving.

Finding out what turns you on
We may all be born with an instinctive or innate response to certain stimuli – it may be something as simple as certain rounded shapes.

'We don't yet know, this is just an idea,' says Amsterdam researcher Dr Laan. 'But we do know that the sexual system needs a stimulus of some kind.' She wants to study our response in the brain to certain stimulating objects to try to define whether some things are more stimulating than others – and what they are. 'I do think that the sexual system is activated as a result of internal and external factors. But sometimes we may not be aware of what that stimulus is.' It is worth people finding out about their own personal triggers, she believes. The advice is 'don't be afraid of fantasy or sexual imagery' if it turns you on.

Couples in a long-term relationship can get so used to the same stimulus that they no longer get turned on by their partner, which may be why so many older women in long-term relationships complain of a loss of desire or libido, and blame it all on the menopause. 'It is much easier to think you have a lack of testosterone or you have some kind of disease which is causing this rather than admit that your partner no longer sexually excites you.'

What to do about it
- you could try more adventurous sex with your partner. This takes courage and good communication and it will only work if you are both happy to try
- learn how to fantasise and use sexual imagery (see *chapter twelve – fantasy and lovemaking techniques*).

Research by Dr Beverly Whipple has shown:
- that women can experience orgasm through imagery alone
- that their physiological response to orgasm and the 'feeling' of orgasm is the same as that achieved through genital stimulation

Learn about self-stimulation
This can help you understand more about your body and your own sexual responses.

Be relaxed about it. And take your time. It's probably best to do these exercises in your bedroom, so you can lie comfortably but make sure the room is pleasantly warm. A warm bath can help. Then, lie on the bed and gently massage your body. You might choose to use an unperfumed massage oil. Start with the arms and legs, then move on to your chest and abdomen. At this stage, the breasts and genitals are out of bounds.

Now gently move around your breasts, use stroking rather than pummelling. Circle your nipple, one at a time and feel the sensations you experience. When you feel really relaxed, move on to the genitalia. Try altering the amount of pressure you apply – from lighter touches to fairly firm pressure. Now concentrate on the front part of your vulva and the hair area over the pubis. Again, experiment with different types of massage movements.

You will probably feel the pencil-like structure, the body of your clitoris. Concentrate massage on this and move your massaging fingers up and down and across this structure. You should be able to identify the type of touch and the amount of pressure that gives you the most response.

Remember the object of the exercise so far is to feel the sensation you get, not to become sexually aroused. This is really an exercise to get used to the different feelings you experience with each part of your body and with the different techniques used. You may also like to explore the sensuality of the vagina by inserting a finger. Make sure you are well-lubricated, then gently probe the area, especially the front wall. You may find an exceptionally sensitive region, the G-spot. Try varying the amount of pressure you apply (this may give you the feeling you need the loo). If you don't become sexually aroused, try thinking about images or experiences you've had in the past that you've found arousing. This should give you a better idea of what you do or don't find stimulating. Then you can then pass the knowledge on to your partner.

Learn to let go

'Sex is not the be all and end all for me, but my husband sees it as an equal part of everything else. I may have changed my opinion because of a lack of desire – when things are good I do feel it's making a difference. It enhances things, there is less tension and we are more relaxed. When it's good I do enjoy it – it's just (the problem of) getting there.'
Michaela, aged 35.

Women who experience orgasm problems invariably have an inability to let go, to take that extra step and momentarily lose control at orgasm. One of your goals should be reducing tension. The relaxation techniques outlined above and in other parts of this book will help. But you may also find it helpful to talk over a self-pleasuring programme with a sex therapist.

One of the keys to being able to let go is feeling good about yourself, which may mean coming to terms with imperfections in your body. It can be difficult to change this way of thinking. If you feel bad about your genitals try looking at them in a mirror and do this until you feel comfortable with the way you are.

A therapist will explain that you are fundamentally responsible for your own orgasms – so there is no point blaming your partner. This creates a cycle of anger or dissatisfaction plus feelings of guilt and these emotions are more likely to trigger sexual aversion. You are the one who needs to know what turns you on and what you enjoy, in terms of being touched and caressed.

Sex and poor health – getting over the fears

It is possible to enjoy sex after a heart attack and after major surgery if the emphasis is on intimacy and gentleness and understanding the partner's needs. Many people who have had heart attacks worry that sex will trigger another one, but the risk is low. The British Heart Foundation says sex can be resumed three weeks after a heart attack, but talk to your doctor first.

Having a hysterectomy can influence self-esteem but as long as the operation is performed correctly with attention paid to the nerves in the pelvic region a hysterectomy will not take away the ability to enjoy sex. (Talk to your gynaecologist about any concerns).

Some women may feel less feminine after hysterectomy and could benefit from counselling (see *chapter four – sex and the mind*).

The same feelings may apply if you have had a mastectomy or a lumpectomy: your confidence at remaining a sexual partner is bound to be affected. You will need to get your fears, worries and feelings out into the open. You will need time to mourn the loss of your breast and your partner may also need help to adjust. Don't hide yourself from your partner, he will need to confront the loss.

These days many women opt for reconstruction. This can be done well after the initial surgery. If you think this would help regain your sexual confidence, discuss the pros and cons with a breast care nurse, your oncologist or surgeon.

Arthritis is a crippling and painful condition: and sometimes the drugs given to relieve the problems can affect sexual function. Use heat to relax – warm baths, rest, and massage. You may want to explore different, more comfortable positions for sex to relieve painful areas of the body. Use cushions and soft throws to help make the area for lovemaking more comfortable. Place cushions under the hips and ask your partner to lie in a T-position with his legs across or under you rather than lying with his weight on top of you.

Prolapse of the womb can affect your sex life. You may experience a dragging sensation, discomfort and also embarrassing incontinence. Prolapse can be corrected with surgery which involves taking a tuck in the front and rear walls of the vagina: discuss any worries about the consequences on your sex life – it may actually improve your ability to grip the penis and also help incontinence problems.

11

adjustments to your sex life

Sexual problems tend to come in waves and cycles. There are times in our lives when our sexual desire for a partner wanes, or the desire has been switched off because of a partner's potency problems.

The problem with sex is that once you have neglected it for a while you may find it hard to become interested again. This may be a consequence of childbirth. You may have been put off sex at the end of pregnancy because you felt large or uncomfortable. Sometimes it may have been because your partner had an unwarranted fear that he might hurt the baby so your sex life had cooled off.

Bereavement, the diagnosis of a serious illness, worries about your child's behaviour, a sick child or a sick partner can all directly influence our sex lives. Sex may become much less of a priority, and if the problem is long-term this can also lead to a long-term lack of interest and a lack of desire which effectively needs to be restored, and gently, compassionately, rekindled when you feel ready.

Many women whose partners had been impotent for years but who have been helped with Viagra or other treatments for erectile dysfunction, have called the Sexual Dysfunction Association helpline, unsure and anxious about coping with a radical change in their sex lives. As a result the association is urging doctors involved in treating impotent men to involve the partner from the beginning.

In this chapter I explore:
- sex after childbirth
- balancing the demands of modern life with sexuality
- sex again after impotency

Sex after childbirth

This is a time when you may not want sex because you are tired, stressed, emotionally bound-up with the baby with little room for your partner, and you have to cope with an altered body shape. Research suggests that in many cases it can take women up to a year to return to the level of sexual activity and enjoyment they had before having a baby. And one of the biggest problems is thought to be painful intercourse – around 70% of women are believed to suffer this. Painful sex after childbirth is sometimes associated with a psychological barrier after a particularly long or painful birth or one which is very invasive – when a doctor may have used forceps or a woman has undergone vaginal examinations she was not comfortable with.

Changes in sexuality begin long before the birth: as you change shape and become more maternal, there may be mixed feelings towards your own sexuality. After the birth, the new role of 'mother' has to sit comfortably with the part of yourself which is also a 'lover'. Getting used to your altered body image takes time: you may feel alienated from your body and this may express itself as a lack of sexual interest. You may need extra help to get over this hurdle. All this can be made worse by overwhelming tiredness and disturbed sleep.

But the change is not purely psychological – there are an array of physiological changes caused by circulating hormones and stretched muscles. The pelvic floor may well be weakened leading to temporary incontinence and there may be pain from episiotomies: both can put women off sex. The pain of vaginal tears can have long-lasting psychological consequences which might need addressing if sex is not resumed within six to eight weeks after the birth.

Research by John Bancroft, senior research fellow at the Kinsey Institute in America, found a difference in sexual arousal and interest between breast- and bottle-feeding mothers. A breastfeeding woman whose prolactin levels remain high and whose ovarian function is suppressed has a different hormonal profile to the bottle-feeding mother, he found.

Prolactin inhibits oestrogen production which in turn will affect vaginal lubrication leading to discomfort and pain just as a menopausal woman might experience. It is believed that persistent or long-term breastfeeders may experience a lack of sexual interest and enjoyment and pain on intercourse.

This might be because of:
- greater interruption of sleep
- pain through episiotomies
- low androgen levels
- low oestrogen levels affecting vaginal cells

Self-help

- look in a mirror to examine genitals. Scar tissue or tears may not be as bad as you imagined and wounds may be smaller
- don't delay intercourse too long after childbirth – six to eight weeks is about right. On the other hand don't allow your partner to pressurise you into intercourse until you feel you are ready.
- find other loving ways to be intimate – like holding, hugging and touching
- seek specialist help if you think your problem may be linked to post-natal depression
- try to set time aside for your partner. He may feel left out if you become intensely wrapped up in the new baby.
- do Kegel's exercises to straighten pelvic floor (see *page 125*)
- ensure you and your partner enjoy some form of relaxation therapy together (see *chapter ten – the happiness factor*)
- alternatively, try the 'stimulation therapy' mentioned on page 42 – you could find that an exciting video may do the trick and provide the right physiological starting point for sex

---

HOW BIRTH AFFECTS SEX

Sheila Kitzinger summed up some of the problems in her book, *Woman's Experience of Sex* (Penguin). 'When the birth has been difficult she may be really frightened of and alienated from her body and alarmed by the changes that have been forced on it. 'I felt I might tear at any moment', 'after the poking and prodding I wanted time to recover and have my body to myself again'. She wonders whether she will ever be able to feel that it is hers again to experience with sexual delight. She may be bruised, and sore, and when she shifts from one buttock to the other the stitches in her perineum make her think she is sitting on embedded thorns or slivers of glass.'

A high-tech labour may influence how you feel about your body after birth; if all control is taken from you, you may feel alienated from your body and need help to restore your confidence in it, and to be able to draw pleasure from it. There are fears to overcome: after the delivery; some women shy away from their partner's sexual advances because they associate vagina with birth rather than vagina with pleasure.

Sheila Kitzinger suggests this lovemaking technique. 'Fear that you are going to have pain is very likely to make you tense up inside which then causes a constriction which causes you further pain. So it is important to be able to release your pelvic floor muscles and make them soft, loose and velvety as your partner comes in. Some men think the only way to penetrate is to push. This is not so. If a man has a strong erection he should be able to wait at the entrance to the vagina (with) only the tip of his penis between the outer folds of your labia and you come down to meet him with your muscles. You will discover when you have bulged the muscles out you can then make little movements with them, alternately contracting and releasing so that you stroke him lightly. He avoids all thrusting and leaves the action to you.'

Lovemaking after the birth

The perineum may be very sensitive and sore after birth especially with an episiotomy. Talk to your midwife beforehand about your thoughts on episiotomy versus a tear. Sometimes tears can painful.

- use a gel moisturising lotion to help smooth the way for more comfortable intercourse
- place your hips on cushions so that there is no pressure on your back; you may be more comfortable on top – you have more control over penetration this way
- if you have had a Caesarean section it will be important for your partner not to press down on the scar. Use positions where this is avoided such as rear entry intercourse or lying together in a spoons position.
- if you are breast feeding ask your partner not to put much pressure on your breasts. Some women have problems coming to terms with their breasts as sexually stimulating while they are breast feeding. This is quite normal but you will need to discuss your feelings with your partner.
- explore the vaginal area yourself before you embark on intercourse to find out what feels comfortable and what feels sore. Communicate this to your partner.

Resuming sex with an impotent man

If your partner has had problems with erectile dysfunction, but has had his potency restored with drugs or one of the other treatments now available, the new and possibly high demands for sex may be of particular concern. His potency may have been restored without you knowing about it and without your opinion being sought: doctors report that men frequently come alone to impotence clinics and exclude their partners. One sex therapist said she knew of marriages which had broken up following the prescription of Viagra.

After months or possibly even years of living with impotence, it can take a great deal of adjustment to cope with sex again on a far more regular basis than you have may have been used to for a long time. During that time your body may have changed and you may need extra help and stimulation from your partner to get you in the mood for sex. However, facing a re-launch of your sex life can be worrying and off putting and may not even be desired.

But if you bottle up your feelings believing yourself to be selfish or cold-hearted if you do not succumb to sex, this can lead to problems with vaginal dryness or other physical problems associated with anxiety and lack of desire or sex drive. It becomes a vicious circle: dread or fear of sex, deterioration of relationship, and eventually a possibly breakdown in the partnership.

Much has been written about how great it is for men to have their potency restored with the new impotence treatments which include injections, pumps and tablets. It is thought that between 70 to 90% of men affected by erectile dysfunction can be helped. But there is concern that little thought has been given to the women who may have not had sex with their partner for years.

'Suddenly some women are being faced with an erection after 10 or 15 years without sex,' says Victoria Lehman, a sex therapist with the SDA. 'And it can be quite worrying.' The association would like to see more doctors involving female partners in erectile dysfunction consultations, so that the woman's perspective on the new situation can be openly expressed, allowing any fears and anxieties to be taken into account. Victoria says at present many men seek treatment alone, and sometimes without telling their partner. This could cause great problems within a relationship.

'A woman can face many concerns. Such as if he can do this with me he can do this now with someone else? There may be fears of pregnancy and also of pain on intercourse.

'After years of not having sex a woman may find it uncomfortable especially if she has experienced thinning of the vaginal walls. How can a woman say no comfortably to a partner who has had his potency restored? These issues have not been addressed and they are causing women anxiety.'

Women may have fallen into a comfortable way of life with an impotent man, still enjoying intimacy, cuddles or even orgasm without penetrative sex. Getting used to demands for penetrative sex – possibly frequent demands – can be unwelcome for some, says Lehman. Ideally there needs to be communication between the couple, and some discussion of the potential problems with the prescribing doctor. 'A lot of women have not had sex for many years in this situation and it can all be a bit of a shock after 20 years – we need doctors, and their patients, to open their eyes to this,' she adds.

A woman may have added problems such as fears of losing her newly-potent partner, fears that he may not fancy her sexually any more, or worries that he might die as a result of taking drugs for ED. 'It is so important to talk to women rather than assume that they feel good about their partners having erections again.'

Balancing sexuality with modern life

Modern women are faced with more roles and responsibilities than ever before. Women have fought long and hard for equality but it frequently feels as though everything is horribly out of balance. Not only are we pursuing careers, but also nurturing children and trying to be a responsible parent with time to give, for listening, playing, guiding.

Even if you buy in help such as a nanny or au pair you are still needed to be available as a taxi driver to children's numerous social events, and to be around when a child is sick. There may be extra responsibilities such as looking after an ageing or dying parent or helping out with a partner's problems. You have to fit in time for exercise, shopping, and spending time with friends. You are probably coping with this huge load without the back-up of an extended family. Today we frequently live away from our families and don't have a network of support.

All these demands pressurise our time and sap our energy levels. Sometimes a partner reaching out expecting sex last thing at night is simply the last straw. You feel you have given out all day long and just want some time to yourself, albeit five minutes, before sleep takes over. At these times sex becomes much less of a priority, especially if you normally have sex at bedtime.

Scientists in Quebec have confirmed that career women who juggle difficult jobs with a family face greater risk of stress-related illnesses than their male partners. These women were more likely to have high blood pressure if they had at least two children

A frantic, busy life can only benefit from some radical reappraisal. You may need to ask your partner to help share the load, or encourage teenage children to take more responsibility for themselves. Adapting and changing to suit the situation is something we do in other areas of life when we change jobs or retire. Why not adapt and change in just the same way with a commitment to an improved sex life? We probably don't try this because most of us find it hard to discuss our problems openly. It takes courage to address this area of life but if you can summon it, the rewards will be great.

The starting point is finding more time for your partner. The next step is understanding how your sex lives might have changed from the first flush of romance and especially after having children. 'Sex at 40 will be different from sex at 20,' says Lehman. 'What relationships under pressure might benefit from is a change in attitude.'

Focusing on the importance of intimacy, ensuring you spend time alone together, and understanding the health-giving benefits of a fulfilling and regular sex life (physically and mentally) are all important. Sex doesn't always have to be a long drawn-out process: a 'quickie' can be just as stimulating – as long as you are both aroused enough to participate fully. Sex can actually relieve some of the pressure we are under; it has been shown to reduce stress levels and reduce anxiety. Sex triggers hormones which encourage a closer bonding with our partner.

'The problem is that we all have high standards and expectations. If something is broken we won't hang around, we'll leave the situation or move on,' says Lehman.

Finding time for intimacy is your key to improved sexuality and it is possible to work into a busy schedule: you just need the commitment to do it. It may only need some small, simple actions like switching off the TV and going to bed with each other instead. Or making space in your diary to spend the time with your partner rather than rushing off to the gym or to your separate leisure activities.

By working on maintaining the central relationship in your life and not allowing it to drift because you are under pressure, you may find that an improved sex life follows quite naturally. But it may take planning, care, and nurturing. Above all it takes commitment from each other to make things better.

12

fantasy and lovemaking techniques

In the third chapter (sex and physiology) the known areas providing sexual pleasure are listed. If your sex life is proving less than satisfactory you may want to experiment with new sexual positions to stimulate these areas. This may involve your partner penetrating from a different angle, or gently stimulating your P-spot or G-spot during foreplay. Every woman is individual and you also need to know what stimulates you – and then have the courage to talk it through with your partner.

Talking about sexual response involves honesty and trust: it gets easier after the first attempts. Many women find they don't have the words. Use your own words and private signals to express how you feel and what pleases you sexually: this on its own can really help to develop a bond.

- learn about what pleases you, rather than go along with what you have always done. Masturbation and self-pleasuring may not appeal to everyone but many sex therapists recommend it as a way of discovering what arouses you as an individual.
- examine psychological 'blocks'. Prof. Alan Riley believes that women are governed far more by psychological influences than men. Any conflict can immediately block arousal. If you are stressed or have had a bad day or feel angry and upset at your partner, your feelings will influence your sexual arousal in the evening. If, on the other hand, you have had a good, fulfilling and satisfactory day you will be far more in the mood for love.
- many women experience 'reflected desire' – they get turned on by their partner's desire for them. US researchers have found that women respond to being desired and thought of as attractive and sexy – and then being told about it. Encourage compliments from your partner and explain you need to feel loved and admired.

- consider your sexual compatibility. Some women who think they have no sex drive may in fact simply have a low sex drive which is normal for them. But this sex drive may become suffocated by a partner who wants sex more often than his partner. One way to find out is to abstain from sex for one or two weeks, but keep a diary noting when you feel sexy and when your partner does. You may find that, with the pressure for sex off for a fortnight, you are feeling very sexy by day 12. Then it is a matter of compromise: once your partner understands your sex drive and you understand his you should strive to find a middle course so that you are both satisfied and the pressure for sex is removed.

- over-familiarisation can be a passion killer. Long-term relationships become flooded with non-sexual concerns which wipe out the sexual spark. Ensure you each have your own space and respect your time alone, making times spent together special. This is much harder for couples who work and live together but it is something worth considering if you find you lack the desire you once had for each other. You will need to work out how to get around this on your own terms in a way to suit you both. Try to vary the time and place you make love rather than the same night, the same time and in the same position.

- consider viewing some sexy movies together. Some companies now make videos specifically for women, by women. These erotic films are often used therapeutically by sex clinics who want to study arousal problems.

- if films are not your scene try reading some arousing books just before bed. Women's top shelf books are growing in popularity and are very easy to get hold of. Women often find they are turned on by words in a book followed by advances from their partner.

- take time to ask your partner about their likes and dislikes. Be interested as well as interesting; this helps build a satisfying and fulfilling relationship. Most people find that sex is really fulfilling when there is trust and communication and a sense of contentment with each other.

- use your friends as a sounding board: girlie nights talking about sex problems can be really therapeutic and are a useful time to offload. Your problems may not seem so frightening when you hear what others are going through. Friends like to talk about their sexuality and sensuality – use this positive outlet.

- try to become more pleasure than goal-orientated. Don't assume that sexual activity has to end in penetrative sex and orgasm. This puts pressure on you and your partner to perform. Rather, view each aspect of intimacy such as kissing or holding as an entity in its own right not necessarily leading on to any next stage.

Fantasy is an important part of a sex life: but some women maintain they cannot and do not fantasise at all. In one survey only 50% of women said they fantasise while making love. Don't be put off by the word 'fantasy'. If you can daydream then you can fantasise.

Betty Dodson says in her book *Sex for One* it had never dawned on her to use her mind for sexual content until she was 36 and a lover began to arouse her with his sexual fantasies, fuelled by his imagination. Dodson says she began to develop and expand her fantasy world by replaying a 'hot sexual experience'. Sometimes it was a recent experience and sometimes she would change a few details. But it was reading books and magazines which helped her most. However, she also discovered that simply looking at attractive men in a magazine did not do the trick: she says she needed some kind of emotional or intellectual interaction to inspire the desire.

In her book she lists the sexual fantasy scenarios which are most popular. These include:

- playing doctor
- being made to perform sexually against your will
- being punished or humiliated
- getting strip searched
- having sex with a football team or other 'gang bang' scenes

There is no certification of fantasies: they can be as far-fetched as you like. Research has shown that women's fantasies change with the times. Whereas women once fantasised about being raped, today it is more likely that women fantasise about overpowering a man. Experts in the field of sexual fantasy say that women have changed from imagining the submissive role in their fantasies to a more dominant one.

You can find out more information about fantasies by reading the books of American author Nancy Friday. She first wrote *My Secret Garden* in 1974 and it lists the fantasies of many women – from rape scenes to those involving submission or humiliation. Her later books, written in the 1990s, show how women's fantasies have moved on – women have become more empowered in their lives and also in their sexual thoughts and daydreams.

Some women find classic romantic notions are the greatest turn-on – think of the numbers of Mills and Boon books which are still read by millions of women. But once again story lines have changed. Rather than women being seen as being seduced they are now the ones to remove the men's clothing, to take control, being active rather than passive active in their sexual fantasy.

However, acting on a fantasy can require the permission of a participating partner. Fantasising about bondage or seducing a man is fine, but if you actually use any of these techniques then you must also have an escape route – a way out. Try using code words or signals which mean 'that's enough'. It keeps this type of sexual activity safe as well as keeping the lines of communication and reality open.

Fantasies allow people to experience situations and pleasures they normally may not find accessible or which may not be socially acceptable. They can help prepare you for sexual intercourse with your partner by using the imagination to help with the sexual arousal process. Mentally rehearsing sexual situations without guilt may pave the way for an improved sexual response and improved sexual feelings particularly if your problem is one of slow arousal – or you are able to become sexually aroused, but it takes time.

Useful aids

- *My Secret Garden: Women's Sexual Fantasies*, Quartet Books, 2001, £8.00
- Look out for films by Candida Royalle. She founded Femme Productions in 1984 in order to create erotic films from a woman's perspective that that could be enjoyed by both women and men. She has made at least 16 films. The Femme line has gone on to win several awards and is now distributed worldwide by Adam & Eve (www.candidaroyalle.com).

The internet has spawned cyber fantasy land: there are interactive online chat rooms in which participants can write out their wildest fantasies without anyone knowing them – or their gender. Fantasies are portrayed in books and films written and produced especially for women and these may help you develop fantasies of your own.

In summary, fantasies reveal what it is that you personally find arousing. You can begin to learn how to fantasise by simply thinking of erotic images and then start to talk about them with your partner. You could ask your partner to reciprocate or encourage him to speak to you in detail about them: he may prefer to do this with the lights dimmed or off, and you lying next to him listening and eventually responding.

Kissing

In long-term relationships kissing is often forgotten: but men and women do find deep prolonged kissing stimulating. Try to recall the early days of your romance and how you enjoyed kissing. Try using it earlier in the day as a signal or prelude to the promise of sex in the evening. Tell your partner where you enjoy being kissed: experiment with different parts of the body, the back, neck, ears, even the feet and toes.

Lots of foreplay

Women who suffer low sexual desire might find it helpful to concentrate on long bouts of foreplay with a partner; many women can reach orgasm with foreplay alone. Ask your partner to take time to explore your external genitalia rather than simply focusing on penetrating the vagina; that, as you will have read earlier, may not be enough to excite you sexually – other surfaces need to be explored, touched, rubbed and caressed. Take some pressure off lovemaking sessions by agreeing with your partner that full intercourse need not happen every time you become intimate. Just lying with your partner, stroking, talking, hugging and kissing each other can sometimes be enough. Tension and tightness of the vagina can happen when there is pressure to perform or take part in vaginal intercourse without the necessary preparation.

Ensure the room is ready for love; with soft lights, aromatherapy vapouriser burning, soft music, plenty of cushions, rugs and covers. Concentrate solely on your partner: clear all thoughts of children and work from your mind.

Foreplay can include undressing each other, touching each other in the genital area and all over the body, kissing, oral sex – gentleness and lightness of touch should be the key words at this stage. This approach will help to relax you and also helps you to enjoy feeling wanted and desired without the pressure of full, thrusting and possibly painful intercourse. After prolonged foreplay you may feel lubricated enough to want to make love and you may then be ready for more dynamic thrusting.

Masturbation – or 'self-loving'

You are unlikely to have an orgasm if you have negative feelings about your partner – including anger, sadness or bitterness. These conflicts may need to be resolved before you can let go again with your partner.

The next step is discovering what turns you on: you may need to learn how to masturbate and a good therapist will provide you with information about how to do this if you have never masturbated before.

You will be reassured that it is not 'dirty' or 'abnormal' and you may need this reassurance if you were discouraged from touching yourself as a child. Some women find this idea distasteful or embarrassing to discuss but remember that your genitals belong to you. Your partner will not magically or telepathically know what to do but if you explore yourself and find out what is pleasurable you will be able to communicate this to him later. You need to know what turns you on in order to tell your partner. Ensure you have your own space and private time to explore your body. Some women masturbate regularly and climax without the distractions of a partner. This is entirely normal. Some therapists recommend sexual fantasising to help women masturbate and reach a climax.

Try some of the suggestions above but remember that open communication with your partner, which includes explaining just how you feel, and what you like during sex, will help to improve your sexual relationship and fulfillment. It does take courage, especially if you have been unable to talk openly before and you may need specialist help to see you through until you gain confidence.

John Bancroft in his book *Human Sexuality and Its Problems* explains that you will benefit from indulging in some healthy pampering, listening to good music, reading interesting, erotic literature, looking at pictures and enjoying nice smells.

In a self-exploration programme you will be encouraged to explore your own genitalia using a mirror. It is surprising how little women know about their own genitals or prefer not to know. Self-exploration can lead on to gentle genital caressing – fears of loss of control and of masturbation may appear at this stage – but it provides an opportunity to identify the time these feelings appear which can be talked about later with a therapist or your partner.

Masturbation is all about knowing yourself – and discovering what gives you pleasure. If you don't know then you can't tell a partner. This can lead to unsatisfactory sex or a loss of desire for sex. Many women feel uncomfortable about self-discovery or self-pleasuring. You may feel embarrassed or silly: but take your time and you may find it very instructive and helpful. It may help to watch a sexy video or read a book first or during masturbation.

Start by stroking the genitals and gently touching the clitoris, discovering its position. You may find a little lubrication helps. Concentrate on stimulating rather than rubbing the clitoris – rubbing can actually be quite painful. Slip a finger inside the vagina and see if you enjoy the sensation from different angles. You may find some sensitive or dry areas you could tell your partner about.

Inside the vagina between the urethra and front wall of the vagina is the G-spot: but don't worry if you can't feel anything. Not every woman can. You may want to try bringing yourself to orgasm, possibly using fantasy.

Sexual techniques

CHANGE POSITIONS

Finding out what pleases you should be fun – and exciting. But you will need to be able to talk to your partner and be willing to try different techniques with the aim of restoring sexual dynamism in your relationship. This might be difficult at first but keep trying – it really could help to improve the quality of your sex life.

Changing your lovemaking positions may be the trigger to improving your desire if your problem is one of a long-term relationship and fading libido. You may find that your erogenous zones are not being aroused – they are being ignored. You may have become quite bored with the routine of being on top or underneath. The missionary position with the woman underneath and the man on top can make you feel trapped or squashed, although it is ideal for kissing and talking to each other.

This position may not be ideal for stimulation of the G-spot or the P-spot. You can ring the changes by wrapping legs around your partner's waist or even over his shoulders.

For deeper penetration in the missionary position, pull your knees right up to your chest then place your legs over your partner's back so that the penis jostles against the enlarged urethra. You may have to move about quite considerably to find the 'right' position in which you enjoy the best stimulation.

Alternatively, sit upright and astride your partner, or sit up facing each other. Being on top can be erotic for women and offers greater freedom of movement than lying underneath the partner. Use the techniques outlined above of fantasy and masturbation. Take control by moving your partner's hand into the most arousing position.

Many women say that being on top is more stimulating: because they are able to

TIPS

■ ask your partner to tell you what he likes and loves about you
■ if it helps, have a glass of wine before lovemaking. Take care, however, as too much will adversely affect your ability to make love
■ learn to become more intimate with your partner.
■ talk more to each other, kiss, hold, touch and hug each other and confide your fears more to each other. Sex promotes the release of oxytocin, a chemical which helps bonding between sexual partners

control the amount of clitoral stimulation more accurately. Strategically place pillows under hips to raise the genital area for a different form of sensation. Lying face to face is another gentle way of making love. – it can be very comfortable and loving and allows you to touch your partner easily. If one partner places their leg over the other it will help to bind you together. The spoons position with the man lying behind, is often considered a good way of stimulating the G-spot. If you are feeling exhausted the T-position is helpful: you lie over your partner who lies on his side. Here you control the movement by gently rocking. Above all ensure you are warm, and comfortable.

CHANGE LOCATION
If you are very much a bedroom couple, consider changing the location: from the bedroom to the bathroom for instance (lit by candles, a warm bubble bath). Even making love on the floor can generate different sensations.

CHANGE THE TIMING
Think about the timing of sex: rather than the usual night-time routine, have an early morning shower and snuggle back into bed with each other. Switch off the TV and go to bed instead.

USE SEX AIDS
Sex aids can be fun if you both want to try. A vibrator is the most common sex toy available and you can both try using it to stimulate different parts of the body. Sex aids may not dramatically change your sex life but may help to enhance it or introduce a different element of excitement.

Remember: it is your right to seek a healthy, fulfilling sex life. And having a fulfilling intimate life can reflect on the rest of your life in a very positive way. It is also your right to seek help when things go wrong.

The last word . . . why sex is good for you
Dr David Weeks, the head of Old Age Psychology at the Royal Edinburgh Hospital, spent more than 10 years studying a group of 3,500 people in the UK and America who are

considered to be 'super young'. These are people who look, act and often feel far younger than their chronological age. One of his key findings is that the people identified as super young tended to have sex more often – there is, he reports 'lots of great sex in the context of mature, mutually shared erotic unions.'

He says that 'in all my years as a clinical psychologist I've never encountered a group of men or women in which there was such a healthy, robust romantic life – and I see many normal, well-adjusted people in my research. By any standard the super young have a remarkably well-developed ability to communicate with their partners and to empathise with one another with great delight which accounts for the greater stability and rich rewards of their relationship.'

Improving the quality of your sex life, advises Dr Weeks, can help make you look between four and seven years younger. He has found that a good sex life can reduce stress and lead to greater contentment.

With an orgasm the body feels good – sex releases a group of substances in the brain, among them beta endorphins, natural painkillers which also alleviate anxiety. Sex also triggers the release of human growth hormone which acts, through another group of peptide hormone substances, to reduce fatty tissues and increase lean muscle in various parts of the body 'giving a more youthful appearance.' Dr Weeks' study also found that sex stimulates the immune system – perhaps by as much as 20%.

During orgasm women produce oxytocin which acts upon the emotional centre of the brain. It plays a part in the nurturing, maternal behaviour – and, says Dr Weeks, 'a lover who regularly stimulates his mate's oxytocin will be rewarded with warmer feelings of affection'. This intense mutual pleasure increases bonding. 'Ongoing sexual frustration probably has an equal and opposite effect: most marriages that crack up are preceded by a decline in the rate of female orgasm.'

More reasons why sex is good for you:

Sexually active people are off work less according to research by the Advanced Study of Human Sexuality in San Francisco. Sex could regulate hormone levels. Sex keeps the vagina muscles well exercised to ward off atrophy. Research in the States suggests that women who have more sex have higher levels of oestrogen circulating in the bloodstream – excellent for skin and bone density.

Sex is an excellent way to burn up calories at the rate of four or five a minute, and it can soon add up. To summarise:

- sex may boost the immune system
- sex will reduce feelings of stress and tension
- sex will help promote natural bonding with a partner

Useful further reading

Beat Menopause Naturally by Maryon Stewart, Natural Health Publishing, £9.99

The Phyto Factor by Maryon Stewart, Vermilion, £10.99

Human Sexuality by Masters and Johnson, Longman, £46.99

Regaining Potency, the answer to male impotence by Oliver Gillie, Self-Help Direct, £10.95

What Really Works in Natural Health: The Only Guide You'll Ever Need by Susan Clark, Bantam Press, £10.99

Nutrients A-7: A User's Guide to Foods, Herbs, Vitamins, Minerals and Supplements by Michael Sharon, Carlton Books Ltd., £10.99

The Relate Guide to Sex in Loving Relationships by Sarah Litvinoff, Vermilion, £7.99

On a more light hearted note read:
Once More, With Feeling by Victoria Coren and Charlie Skelton, Fourth Estate £8.99

Acknowledgements

Grateful thanks to all contributors and most importantly to the brave women who have told their stories in order to get the message across to other sufferers.

Special thanks to the following dedicated professionals: Dr Frances Quirk, Dr Kevan Wylie, Ann Tailor, Mary Davern, Jane Roy, Prof. Edward Laumann, Dr John Dean, Malcolm Whitehead, Dr Roy Levin, Prof. Barry Komisaruk, Dr David Nunns, Fabia Brackenbury, Dr David Goldmeier, Ian Russell, Catherine Allen and Christine Lacy